Evidence-Based Herbal and Nutritional Treatments for Anxiety in Psychiatric Disorders

David Camfield • Erica McIntyre
Jerome Sarris
Editors

Evidence-Based Herbal and Nutritional Treatments for Anxiety in Psychiatric Disorders

Editors
David Camfield
School of Psychology
University of Wollongong
Wollongong
New South Wales
Australia

Jerome Sarris
Department of Psychiatry
Faculty of Medicine
The University of Melbourne
Melbourne
Australia

Erica McIntyre
School of Psychology
Charles Sturt University
Bathurst
New South Wales
Australia

ISBN 978-3-319-42305-0 ISBN 978-3-319-42307-4 (eBook)
DOI 10.1007/978-3-319-42307-4

Library of Congress Control Number: 2016958529

Printed on acid-free paper

This Springer imprint is published by Springer Nature
The registered company is Springer International Publishing AG Switzerland
The registered company address is Gewerbestrasse 11, 6330 Cham, Switzerland

For Kath, Jordan and Tyler

DC

For Martin and Monique

"If the person you are talking to does not appear to be listening, be patient. It may simply be that he has a small piece of fluff in his ear." - A.A. Milne, Winnie-the-Pooh

EM

To the Mermaid, the Goblin, and the Leprechaun

Maintenant, je sais ce qu'est l'amour

JS

Foreword

A common theme today across many media articles about herbal and nutritional treatments is there is no valid evidence for their efficacy, and the risk of harm is high due to potential issues such as adulteration (sometimes deliberately with pharmaceutical drugs), idiosyncratic hepatotoxicity, and herb–drug interactions. While the lack of data may have held true three or four decades ago, even a cursory search of the published literature reveals an accumulating evidence of safety and efficacy for such treatments, sometimes in a complementary role with mainstream pharmaceuticals. For example, there are now more than 30 clinical trials on the herb kava (*Piper methysticum*), including several by one of the editors of this text (Jerome Sarris). The clinical research on the psychiatric applications of N-acetylcysteine is particularly promising (as will be outlined in the context of anxiety in Chap. 5).

This growing evidence for herbal treatments is occurring in a landscape of increasing challenges for the use of mainstream drugs in psychiatric disorders. Again, even a cursory review of the literature highlights a few of these. Not the least is the complexity of the modern patient and our increasing understanding of the many factors involved in such conditions. Taking depression as one example, one review highlighted that there are now more than five plausible hypotheses of the cause of depression, with the likelihood that these aetiological factors interact with each other in unique and complex ways in the individual patient [1]. Hence 'a one size fits all' approach to depression, especially using a single pharmaceutical intervention, might see many patients miss out on optimal treatment. It should be no surprise therefore that the numbers needed to treat (NNTs) for a single patient to respond to a selective serotonin reuptake inhibitor (SSRI) can be as high as 12 [2]. Another review concluded that 'Although recent work suggests that cognitive impairment is a treatable component of major depressive disorder, and regulatory agencies seem to be encouraging treatment development for this indication, existing treatments do little to return patients level of cognitive performance to normal' [3]. Hence, Chap. 4 on cognitive anxiolytics is a timely contribution to the debate, as is Chap. 6 on herbal and nutritional treatments for comorbid anxiety and mood disorders.

But there are other looming problems. One example is the renewed concerns over the safety of SSRIs in teenagers, which are used to manage both anxiety and mood disorders. A reanalysis of a decade-old trial on paroxetine and imipramine in adolescence found no evidence of benefit over placebo, and found, in fact, evidence of harm, including suicidal ideation and behaviour [4]. The authors concluded that 'The extent of the clinically significant increases in adverse events in the paroxetine and imipramine arms, including serious, severe, and suicide related adverse events, became apparent only when the data were made available for reanalysis. Researchers and clinicians should recognise the potential biases in published research, including the potential barriers to accurate reporting of harms that we have identified. Regulatory authorities should mandate accessibility of data and protocols'.

Not surprisingly, modern patients are increasingly looking for a third treatment option for their psychiatric problems, and this becomes urgently relevant in the case of children – an option that sits between taking a drug and doing nothing. However, engaging this third option by using herbs and nutraceuticals must be credible; it needs to be underpinned by evidence. On the other hand, it is acknowledged that such agents are gentle and subtle; indeed that is their strength and what renders them valid third options.

How can a pharmacologically mild agent render a clinically relevant outcome? Here enters the new concept of network pharmacology, at least as it applies to medicinal plants. Due to their chemical complexity, even a single herbal extract is a nature-designed multi-agent medicine that can simultaneously target a range of pharmacological effects. This helps to explain why identifying the 'active constituent' in many herbal extracts has proved to be so difficult. For most if not all herbal extracts, the 'active constituent' is the whole extract itself, as illustrated by research on the antidepressant activity of St John's wort. The potential for chemical complexity to confer polyvalent activity or polypharmacology can also explain the apparent therapeutic versatility of herbal extracts.

In a review, Gertsch observed that herbal extracts might in fact be 'intelligent mixtures' of secondary plant metabolites that have been shaped by evolutionary pressures. As such, they could represent complex therapeutic mixtures possessing an inherent and coherent synergy and polyvalence. Gertsch also notes that another important concept related to polyvalence is that of network pharmacology, as originally proposed by Hopkins. In the context of plant extracts (which, for commonly used herbs as described in this book, typically contain hundreds of potentially bioactive natural products with only mild activity), it is possible that different proteins within the same signalling network are only weakly targeted. However, this is sufficient to shut down or activate a whole pathway by network pharmacology. In other words, network pharmacology can explain how a number of weakly active plant secondary metabolites in an extract may be sufficient to exert a potent pharmacological effect without the presence of a highly bioactive compound. In the context of herbal network pharmacology, Paul Ehrlich's concept of the magic bullet is supplanted by one of a 'green shotgun', to paraphrase Gertsch and James Duke.

The authors of this book have responded admirably to the considerable challenge of reviewing the current evidence that supports the role of herbal and nutritional treatments for anxiety (including anxiety comorbid with depression). They are well published in the field, including a recent survey of herbal medicine use behaviour in Australian adults experiencing anxiety [5]. The high level of self-prescribing discovered is of significant concern in terms of both adequate treatment and potential herb–drug interactions. It highlights that clinicians of all persuasions need to be better informed on this topic. What better resource is available then than this comprehensive text that, through its various chapters, systematically looks at the evidence for and role of herbal anxiolytics, the all-important herbal adaptogens to support stress management, and cognitive anxiolytics (again primarily herbal), together with the key nutraceuticals for anxiety? The ever-pressing issue of herb–drug interactions is covered by a handy table. Above all, the information is informed and supported by the unique blend of research and clinical experience that the authors bring to their work, something that is often lacking in texts from the complementary medicine field.

Kerry Bone
Director Research & Development - MediHerb
Adjunct Professor - School of Applied Clinical Nutrition
New York Chiropractic College, USA

Queensland, Australia

References

1. Dale E, Bang-Andersen B, Sánchez C (2015) Emerging mechanisms and treatments for depression beyond SSRIs and SNRIs. Biochem Pharmacol 2015;95(2):81–97
2. Magni LR, Purgato M, Gastaldon C et al (2013) Fluoxetine versus other types of pharmacotherapy for depression. Cochrane Database Syst Rev 2013;(7):CD004185
3. Keefe RS (2016) Treating cognitive impairment in depression: an unmet need. Lancet Psychiatry 2016;3(5):392–393
4. Le Noury J, Nardo JM, Healy D et al (2015) Restoring Study 329: efficacy and harms of paroxetine and imipramine in treatment of major depression in adolescence. BMJ 2015;351:h4320
5. McIntyre E, Saliba AJ, Wiener KK et al (2016) Herbal medicine use behaviour in Australian adults who experience anxiety: a descriptive study. BMC Complement Altern Med 2016;16(1):60

Acknowledgements

We would like to thank all the people who generously contributed to this book, gave their support to the project and were involved in its production: Rachel Arthur, Richard Brown, Michael Coe, Patricia Gerbarg, Jane Hutchens, Dennis McKenna, David Mischoulon, Naomi Perry, Danielle Mathersul, Genevieve Steiner, Kerry Bone, Con Stough, Rodney Croft, Andrew Scholey, Corinna Schaefer, Geetha Dhandapani and Saanthi Shankhararaman.

Contents

The Need for Evidence-Based Herbal and Nutritional Anxiety Treatments in Psychiatry

1

David A. Camfield, Erica McIntyre, and Jerome Sarris

1.1 The Experience of Anxiety

Anxiety is a ubiquitous part of the human condition, with anxiety disorders suffered by 14.4 % of Australians over a 12-month period [1], and 26.3 % over a lifetime [2]. Similar figures exist for the USA, with a life-time prevalence as high as 33.7 % [3]. Whilst fear is an emotional response to imminent threat, anxiety involves the anticipation of future threat [4] and may be experienced in response to a wide range of circumstances including public speaking, financial stress, separation, traumatic experiences, or substance use [5]. To the individual who is experiencing symptoms of anxiety, it is a distressing psychological state—and one that is associated with both apprehensive thoughts together with physiological symptoms including a

D.A. Camfield (✉)
School of Psychology, University of Wollongong, Wollongong, NSW, Australia

Centre for Human Psychopharmacology, Swinburne University of Technology, Hawthorn, VIC, Australia
e-mail: camfield@uow.edu.au

E. McIntyre
School of Psychology, Charles Sturt University, Bathurst, NSW, Australia

Australian Research Centre in Complementary and Integrative Medicine (ARCCIM), Faculty of Health, University of Technology, Ultimo, NSW, Australia

J. Sarris
University of Melbourne, Department of Psychiatry, The Melbourne Clinic, The Professorial Unit, ARCADIA Mental Health Research Group, 2 Salisbury St, Richmond, Melbourne, VIC 3121, Australia

Centre for Human Psychopharmacology, Swinburne University of Technology, Hawthorn, VIC, Australia

D. Camfield et al. (eds.), *Evidence-Based Herbal and Nutritional Treatments for Anxiety in Psychiatric Disorders*, DOI 10.1007/978-3-319-42307-4_1

pounding heart, difficulties in breathing, nausea and a feeling of detachment from the environment. Further, with chronic anxiety come additional problems such as restlessness, fatigue, difficulties with concentration and sleep, as well as muscular tension. Many individually additionally begin to adversely modify their lifestyles in order to avoid anxiety-provoking situations [6]. Although many individuals will experience transient anxiety as part of their day-to-day life, for other individuals, the symptoms become severe enough to cause significant impairment in day-to-day living. Current first-line treatments for anxiety include pharmaceuticals such as benzodiazepines and serotonin-reuptake inhibitors (SSRIs), as well as cognitive behavioural therapy (CBT) involving exposure to anxiety-provoking stimuli and the targeting of dysfunctional cognitions.

1.2 Limitations of Current Treatment Approaches

Whilst pharmaceutical treatments may be effective in bringing symptomatic relief to some patients, there are known issues which limit their efficacy. First, they do not always work well in conjunction with psychotherapeutic approaches, having been designed as standalone treatments rather than part of an integrative approach. For example, benzodiazepines may limit the efficacy of exposure therapy by blunting the experience of emotional arousal [7]. Antidepressants may also make it more difficult to access emotional states, with feelings of emotional numbness reported by 60 % of participants in a recent survey [8]. Second, many people do not respond to pharmaceutical treatments, with response rates to SSRIs reported at between 60 and 75 % [9]. Third, pharmaceutical treatments have a range of unacceptable side effects, including negative impacts on sexual functioning, appetite and sleep [10–12], and discontinuing treatment can also lead to unwanted side effects and withdrawal symptoms that require careful management [9]. The question of dependency is also pertinent, particularly in the case of tranquilizers and benzodiazepines. But perhaps the greatest issue to contend with is that pharmaceutical treatments for anxiety are often not intended for chronic use, and have not been tested as such in regulatory trials. Whilst more favourable response rates have been shown for CBT in comparison to pharmaceutical anxiety treatments [13–15], cognitive approaches also do not necessarily work for all individuals, particularly in cases where the patient is not 'psychologically minded'.

1.3 Nutritional and Herbal Treatments for Anxiety

As conventional treatments for anxiety are not always effective or suitable for all individuals, it is important to consider other treatment options. As outlined in this book, an evidence-base is building for the efficacy of herbal and nutritional medicines in the treatment of anxiety. This evidence-base is particularly important considering the increasingly widespread use of these substances. For example, it has been estimated that around 34 % of the population in the USA are now using complementary medicines, and similarly 38.4 % of individuals in Australia [16, 17]. The contemporary use of herbal medicine differs significantly from traditional use, as nutraceuticals and herbal extracts are now predominantly commercialized products that are widely accessible [18], and these products are most frequently self-prescribed for anxiety symptoms, in addition to being prescribed by a range of health practitioners [19, 20]. An Australian study of general practitioners found that the majority of doctors did not have the confidence to discuss the use of complementary medicine with their patients as they believed that they lacked the knowledge needed [21]. Another US study found that as little as 20 % of general practitioners were comfortable discussing herbal medicines with their patients [22]. For these reasons, there is a need for greater access to reliable evidence-based information in regards to these substances, both for consumers and health practitioners.

Research conducted so far indicates that there may be some important advantages to the use of nutritional and herbal treatments in contrast to existing treatments. Whilst a majority of pharmaceuticals rely on a single active constituent to deliver therapeutic effects, nutritional substances and herbal extracts typically contain a vast array of psychoactive components [23]. In one regard, this may appear to be a problem for manufacturers wishing to provide a highly standardized treatment, and a simplistic solution may be to try and isolate single active components for extraction. However, any attempt to simplify the complex constellation of chemicals would neglect the fact that synergistic and polyvalent interaction between the components is a key aspect to their therapeutic advantage [24]. The interaction of the various plant components is something that has been well understood in traditional medicinal systems such as Ayurvedic medicine or Traditional Chinese Medicine (TCM) throughout the centuries [25]. Synergism refers to how the therapeutic effect is greater for a combination of substances than would have been expected from a consideration of individual contributions [23]. Polyvalence refers to the inclusion of substances that may not directly contribute to symptom relief, but influence the overall clinical efficacy of the substance; for example, through modification of important processes, including absorption, distribution, metabolism and excretion of bioactive constituents, or by aiding in the reduction of side effects [24]. Many of the natural substances described in this book are excellent examples of synergy and polyvalence; for example, *Salvia* spp., *Valeriana officinalis* and *Hypericum perforatum.*

1.4 Varied Mechanisms of Anxiolytic Actions

Herbal and nutritional treatments for anxiety may exert their effects according to both direct neurotransmitter effects and more chronic cellular effects. It is often the case that each treatment, particularly in the case of herbals, possesses multiple active constituents with sometimes differing and complementary modes of action. In regards to direct neurotransmitter effects, the gamma-aminobutyric acid (GABA) system is often implicated. GABA is the primary inhibitory neurotransmitter in the central nervous system, and also the target of benzodiazepines. Natural substances with known actions on the GABA system include *Piper methysticum* (kava), *Passiflora incarnata* (passionflower), *Matricaria recutita* (chamomile), *Scutellaria lateriflora* (skullcap) and *Valeriana* spp. (valerian); these are typically found to exert sedative as well as anxiolytic effects. Many natural substances have also been found to have effects on serotonin (5-hydroxytryptophan [5-HT]; the biogenic amine that is targeted by antidepressants and is implicated in the regulation of both mood, anxiety and obsessional thinking). Substances with serotonergic mechanisms of action include myo-inositol (MI), *Hypericum perforatum* (St John's wort), *S*-adenosyl methionine (SAMe) and the traditional South American herbal combination Ayahuasca.

In contrast, other substances boost the action of acetylcholine (ACh), a neurotransmitter important for cognitive functioning—these substances include *Bacopa monnieri*, *Ginkgo biloba*, *Salvia* spp. (sage) and *Rosmarinus officinalis* (rosemary). Another class of herbal medicines (adaptogens) aids in adaption to stress, via effects on glucocorticoids and the hypothalamic–pituitary–adrenal (HPA) axis. These medicines have a long history of use in Eastern Europe and Asia, and include *Withania somnifera* (Ashwagandha), *Rhodiolarosea*, *Gotu kola*, *Eleutherococcus senticosus* (Siberian ginseng) and *Schisandra chinensis*. For other natural substances, effects across a number of other neurotransmitter systems have been reported, including glutamate, norepinephrine and dopamine. In addition to direct neurotransmitter effects, perhaps an even greater advantage associated with herbal and nutritional substances is that they exhibit cellular effects that provide overall benefits to brain health, typically in association with chronic use. These include antioxidant and anti-inflammatory effects, endothelial and blood flow effects, together with the lowering of homocysteine (HCy), reduction of beta-amyloid proteins, improved mitochondrial function and the enhancement of neurotrophins (e.g. brain-derived neurotrophic factor) [26].

1.5 Challenges for an Emerging Herbal and Nutraceutical Industry

Notwithstanding the numerous benefits afforded by nutritional and herbal substances, this emerging field of research is still in its infancy. Whilst there is a long history of traditional use associated with several of these substances, in many cases, there are still only a handful of systematic scientific studies which have been conducted to investigate their efficacy in clinical populations. Documented traditional use has guided the therapeutic use of herbal medicines, and informed the focus of further research. In many cases, treating clinicians with an interest in novel treatments have published case studies showing favourable effects observed in their patients. Following reports of clinical effectiveness, open-label studies are typically published, and finally if researchers can secure sufficient funding, then randomized placebo-controlled studies (RCTs) are conducted. It is the latter RCTs which are considered the gold standard regarding evidence of efficacy—and over the past decade, their numbers have been consistently growing.

Another challenge facing researchers, clinicians and consumers related to natural medicines is the current lack of regulatory control. For instance, in Australia, the Therapeutic Goods Administration (TGA) provides a two-tier system of product listing for over-the-counter (non-prescription) health care products. Listed medicines

(AUST L), which are considered to have low-risk ingredients, are assessed for quality and safety but not efficacy (https://www.tga.gov.au/listed-medicines). In contrast, registered medicines (AUST R) are considered to pose a higher level of risk and are required to have comprehensive safety, quality and efficacy data (https://www.tga.gov.au/registered-medicines). Notwithstanding one or two exceptions, complementary and alternative medicines are almost totally absent from the registered medicines list. For this reason, high-quality products may coexist side-by-side with low-quality extracts, and a consumer who wishes to purchase a product such as *Ginkgo biloba* may be led to believe that they are equally as effective. However, it is noteworthy that stricter regulation exists in Europe, with the Medicine and Healthcare Regulatory Agency (MHRA) overseeing the sale of natural products.

Product reliability is an issue that relates to herbal products in particular. The effectiveness of a herbal medicine product can be highly variable. In order to reduce this variability, the concept of phytoequivalence needs consideration, whereby two different types of extracts of the same herb are considered to have the same psychopharmacological effect. Well validated herbal extracts such as *Ginkgo biloba* extract EGb 716 or *Hypericum perforatum* extract LI 160 have been standardized to contain minimum quantities of active ingredients, and are produced according to a protocol which spans from seeding, cultivation, harvesting, drying, extraction, formulation of the dry extract, as well as quality control monitoring [27]. Furthermore, validation studies (RCTs) that have been conducted using standardized extracts only strictly apply to these same extracts. These standardized products ensure a level of phytoequivalence that is more likely to provide a reliable clinical effect.

There are also numerous other important factors which need to be thoroughly investigated and communicated clearly to clinicians and consumers in order to guarantee reliable and valid effects associated with natural products. These issues include: (i) whether the substance is best used acutely and/or chronically, (ii) the effective minimum dose that is required for reliable effects, (iii) the duration of supplementation required (in the case of chronic supplementation), (iv) the time to peak effects (in the case of acute administration), (v) whether the supplement is best used as monotherapy or adjunctive to other treatments, (vi) whether there are any known interactions with common medications, (vii) for which populations are the substances most effective (i.e. non-clinical or clinical) and (viii) for which severity of symptom presentation is the substance most appropriate. These questions are central to determining the conditions associated with therapeutic effects. This is a complex amount of information to navigate; therefore, there needs to be effective translation of this information in order for both clinicians and consumers to make good treatment decisions.

1.6 The Scope of This Book

The aim of the current book is to provide an up-to-date and thorough assessment of the evidence-base regarding herbal and nutritionally based treatments in clinical samples—as well as to present an integrated picture of their routine use in clinical practice. It is intended that the book will be of use to researchers, clinicians and the interested layperson. The focus is on the treatment of DSM-5 anxiety disorders (including panic disorder, agoraphobia, generalized anxiety disorder and social anxiety disorder). Other disorders that typically express high levels of anxiety are also discussed, including obsessive-compulsive and related disorders, together with trauma and stress-related disorders; disorders that were previously subsumed under the anxiety disorders in DSM-IV. Due to the common comorbidity of anxiety and mood disorders, a separate chapter will also be devoted to this topic. Whilst anxiety is also a common feature in psychotic disorders, the treatment of these disorders with natural medicines is beyond the scope of the current book, as there is a current scarcity of research in this area. Finally, the emphasis throughout the book is on the evidence-base regarding single nutritional substances and herbal extracts rather than traditional formulations such as those used in TCM—although this is a worthy topic of discussion in its own right.

Each chapter will consider a different class of herbal or nutritional medicines, categorized primarily according to their psychopharmacological effects (herbal anxiolytics with sedative actions, adaptogens, cognitive anxiolytics, nutritional-based nutraceuticals, treatments for comorbid anxiety and mood disorders, as well as Ayahuasca and other potential anxiolytic phytotherapies, which are emerging treatments in need of further research). The final three chapters of the book are provided by integrative practitioners and herbalists within the field—in order to demonstrate the applied use of these substances in the treatment of patients with often complex presentations of clinically significant anxiety. These chapters provide important insight into the decision-making process around the selection of appropriate combinations of phytotherapies in the treatment of anxiety. Finally, the concluding sections present a list of all known herb–drug interactions. We trust that you find the book to be a valuable and informative contribution to this exciting new field of research and clinical practice.

References

1. Australian Bureau of Statistics. National Survey of Mental Health and Wellbeing: summary of results, 2007. Canberra: ABS; 2007.
2. Slade T et al. 2007 National Survey of Mental Health and Wellbeing: methods and key findings. Aust N Z J Psychiatry. 2009;43(7):594–605.
3. Kessler RC et al. Twelve-month and lifetime prevalence and lifetime morbid risk of anxiety and mood disorders in the United States. Int J Methods Psychiatr Res. 2012;21(3):169–84.
4. Barlow DH. Anxiety and its disorders: the nature and treatment of anxiety and panic. New York: Guilford Press; 1988.
5. Degenhardt L, Topp L. 'Crystal meth' use among polydrug users in Sydney's dance party subculture: characteristics, use patterns and associated harms. Int J Drug Policy. 2003;14(1):17–24.
6. American Psychiatric Association. Diagnostic and statistical manual of mental disorders (DSM-5). 5th ed. Washington, DC: American Psychiatric Association; 2013.
7. Otto MW, McHugh RK, Kantak KM. Combined pharmacotherapy and cognitive-behavioral therapy for anxiety disorders: medication effects, glucocorticoids, and attenuated treatment outcomes. Clin Psychol(Science and Practice). 2010;17(2):91–103.

8. Read J, Cartwright C, Gibson K. Adverse emotional and interpersonal effects reported by 1829 New Zealanders while taking antidepressants. Psychiatry Res. 2014;216(1):67–73.
9. Baldwin D et al. Efficacy of drug treatments for generalised anxiety disorder: systematic review and meta-analysis. BMJ. 2011;342.
10. Serretti A, Chiesa A. Treatment-emergent sexual dysfunction related to antidepressants: a meta-analysis. J Clin Psychopharmacol. 2009;29(3):259–66.
11. Lam RW. Sleep disturbances and depression: a challenge for antidepressants. Int Clin Psychopharmacol. 2006;21(Suppl 1):S25–9.
12. Serretti A, Mandelli L. Antidepressants and body weight: a comprehensive review and meta-analysis. J Clin Psychiatry. 2010;71(10):1259–72.
13. Hofmann SG et al. The efficacy of cognitive behavioral therapy: a review of meta-analyses. Cognit Thera Res. 2012;36(5):427–40.
14. Hofmann SG, Smits JAJ. Cognitive-behavioral therapy for adult anxiety disorders: a meta-analysis of randomized placebo-controlled trials. J Clin Psychiatry. 2008;69(4):621–32.
15. Olatunji BO, Cisler JM, Deacon BJ. Efficacy of cognitive behavioral therapy for anxiety disorders: a review of meta-analytic findings. Psychiatr Clin North Am. 2010;33(3):557–77.
16. Clarke TC, Black LI, Stussman BJ, Barnes PM, Nahin RL. Trends in the Use of Complementary Health Approaches Among Adults: United States, 2002–2012. National health statistics reports. 2015;(79):1–16.
17. Spinks J, Hollingsworth B. Policy implications of complementary and alternative medicine use in Australia: Data from the National Health Survey. The Journal of Alternative and Complement Medicine. 2012;18(4):371–378. http://doi.org/10.1089/acm.2010.0817.
18. Zhang AL et al. A population survey on the use of 24 common medicinal herbs in Australia. Pharmacoepidemiol Drug Saf. 2008;17(10):1006–13.
19. McIntyre E et al. Herbal medicine use behaviour in Australian adults who experience anxiety: a descriptive study. BMC Complement Altern Med. 2016;16:60.
20. McIntyre E et al. Prevalence and predictors of herbal medicine use in adults experiencing anxiety: a critical review of the literature. Adv Intern Med. 2015;2(1):38–48.
21. Pirotta M et al. Complementary medicine in general practice a national survey of GP attitudes and knowledge. Aust Fam Physician. 2010;39:946–50.
22. Zhang Y et al. Discrepancy between patients use of and health providers familiarity with CAM. Patient Educ Couns. 2012;89(3):399–404.
23. Heinrich M et al. Fundamentals of pharmacognosy and phytotherapy. London: Churchill Livingstone; 2004.
24. Williamson EM. Synergy and other interactions in phytomedicines. Phytomedicine. 2001;8:401–9.
25. Bensky D, Gamble A. Chinese herbal formulas. Seattle: Eastland Press; 1991.
26. Camfield DA. Herbal extracts and cognition in adulthood and ageing. In: Riby LM, Smith MA, Foster JK, editors. Nutrition and mental performance – a lifespan perspective. Hampshire, UK: Palgrave Macmillan; 2012.
27. Groot MJ, Van Der Roest J. Quality control in the production chain of herbal products. In: Bogers RJ, Craker LE, Lange D, editors. Medicinal and aromatic plants. The Netherlands: Springer; 2006. p. 253–60.

Part I

Clinical Evidence in Support of Herbal and Nutritional Treatments for Anxiety

Herbal Anxiolytics with Sedative Actions 2

Jerome Sarris and Erica McIntyre

2.1 Introduction

Anxiety disorders such as generalized anxiety disorder (GAD), panic disorder, social phobia, and post-traumatic stress disorder (PTSD) present with a marked element of psychological anxiety and distress [1]. Further, as sleep disorders are highly co-morbid, it is often useful to consider the sedative actions of herbal anxiolytics. Herbal medicines that possess anxiolytic properties generally have effects on gamma-aminobutyric acid (GABA), either via direct receptor binding, ionic channel or cell membrane modulation, GABA transaminase or glutamic acid decarboxylase inhibition. The subsequent increased GABA neurotransmission has a damping effect on stimulatory pathways, which ultimately provides a psychologically calming effect [2]. Mechanisms of action of these phytomedicines have been elucidated via in vitro and in vivo studies. For example, Awad and colleagues [3] sought to determine whether several common herbal medicines directly affected the primary brain enzymes responsible for GABA metabolism. In vitro rat brain homogenate assays revealed aqueous extract of lemon balm (*Melissa officinalis*) to exhibit the greatest inhibition of GABA transaminase activity, while chamomile (*Matricaria recutita*) and hops (*Humulus lupulus*) inhibited glutamic acid decarboxylase activity. In addition

J. Sarris (✉)
University of Melbourne, Department of Psychiatry, The Melbourne Clinic, The Professorial Unit, ARCADIA Mental Health Research Group, 2 Salisbury St, Richmond, Melbourne, VIC 3121, Australia

Centre for Human Psychopharmacology, Swinburne University of Technology, Hawthorn, VIC, Australia
e-mail: jsarris@unimelb.edu.au

E. McIntyre
School of Psychology, Charles Sturt University, Bathurst, NSW, Australia

Australian Research Centre in Complementary and Integrative Medicine (ARCCIM), Faculty of Health, University of Technology, Ultimo, NSW, Australia

D. Camfield et al. (eds.), *Evidence-Based Herbal and Nutritional Treatments for Anxiety in Psychiatric Disorders*, DOI 10.1007/978-3-319-42307-4_2

to treating anxiety disorders, many anxiolytic plant medicines have additional applications, as discussed below in the "clinical considerations" section. The herbs outlined in this section have demonstrated clinical efficacy in treating various types of anxiety disorders, as well as being sedatives. Table 2.1 provides an overview of these herbal medicines.

2.2 Kava (*Piper methysticum*)

2.2.1 Overview

Apart from Kava's (*Piper methysticum*) traditional use for cultural, social, and religious occasions, the plant also has a role as a medicine, and has been used in Western society for its effects on anxiety via physiological and psychological relaxation [4]. It should be noted that while kava is detailed under this section of plants with "sedative actions," this effect is varied, with some consumers potentially experiencing a mentally stimulating effect alongside physiological sedation (due to the combination of GABAergic and noradrenergic effects) [5]. The use of kava has been popularised since the 1990s, with dozens of kava products (of varying quality) being used worldwide for the treatment of anxiety. While selective serotonin re-uptake inhibitors (SSRIs) and benzodiazepines are effective first-line pharmacological treatments of anxiety disorders [6], both agents have unwanted side effects. While there is compelling evidence in support of kava for the treatment of anxiety [7], concerns over hepatotoxicity led to its withdrawal or restriction in many countries since 2002 (overturned by a German court ruling in 2015) [8]. Although not confirmed, reasons for previous liver toxicity may have included: the use of low-quality and inexpensive plant materials (e.g. plant peelings rather than the traditional peeled rhizomes), incorrect use of kava cultivars, and the use of dangerous chemical solvents during extraction [9].

2.2.2 Mechanisms of Action

2.2.2.1 Constituents

The pharmacodynamic anxiolytic mechanism is thought to be attributable to the lipophilic constituents of kava, known as kavalactones [4]. Collectively, kavalactones are concentrated mainly within the rhizomes, roots and root stems of the plant [10, 11]. The distribution of kavalactones progressively decreases towards the aerial parts of the plant [11]. The aerial parts of the plant often contain toxic alkaloids such as piper methystine, and are not used in traditional consumption [12]. Eighteen different kavalactones have been identified to date, with approximately 96 % of the total pharmacological activity attributed to the presence of six kavalactones: methysticin, dihydromethysticin, kavain, dihydrokavain, demethoxy yangonin and yangonin [2, 11].

Several studies have documented a wide spectrum of pharmacological effects of kava including anxiolytic [13], anti-stress [13], sedative [14], analgesic [15], muscle

Table 2.1 Summary of herbal anxiolytics with sedative actions

Herbal medicine	Dosage	Major/active constituents	Key evidence	Potential AEs	Potential clinical use	Clinical advice
Kava (*Piper methysticum*)	Total dose of 50–250 mg of kavalactonesper day, approximating 50–60 mg of kavalactones contained in a tablet	Kavalactones: Formulations higher in kavain and dihydrokavain with lower levels of dihydromethysticin preferred	Mainly positive RCTs and a meta-analysis showing a significant anxiolytic effect over placebo	Very rare potential of liver toxicity; sedation and motor coordination issues at higher doses. High doses and long-term use may cause dermopathy	General anxiety and GAD; potential use in social anxiety; No data on OCD, panic disorder or PTSD (but may have a supportive role); useful for benzodiazepine withdrawal and anxiety presenting with insomnia	Use intermittently and monitor via occasional LFTs if warranted; use recommended dose and avoid co-use with benzodiazepines and alcohol
Passionflower (*Passiflora incarnata*)	Chronic dose: dried herb 1–3 g per day standardized to benzoflavones Acute dose: 500–700 mg standardised to benzoflavones	Benzoflavone, potentially chyrsin	Several positive RCTs showing efficacy in generalised anxiety and preoperative anxiety	Considered quite safe. No interaction found with anaesthetic medication	Generalized anxiety, GAD, preoperative anxiety. No data on OCD, panic disorder, or PTSD; however, may have a supportive role. May be useful for social anxiety given the demonstrated acute effects	A generally safe herbal medicine that can be combined with a range of other anxiolytic and adaptogenic herbal medicines. Monitor adjunctive use with benzodiazepines and SSRIs due to possible potentiation of effect

(continued)

Table 2.1 (continued)

Herbal medicine	Dosage	Major/active constituents	Key evidence	Potential AEs	Potential clinical use	Clinical advice
Chamomile (*Matricaria recutita*)	Dried herb 1–2 g per day standardized to apigenin	Apigenin	An isolated RCT showed efficacy of standardised chamomile in capsule form in GAD	Considered very safe ad commonly used as a tea	GAD and mild anxiety and nervous tension	A generally safe herbal medicine although caution needed for people with *asteracea* plant family allergies
Galphimia (*Galphimia glauca*)	Dried herb 0.6–1 g per day standardized to 0.175–0.348 mg of galphimine B	Galphimine B	Clinical trials showing equivalence to synthetic anxiolytics	No adverse reactions found in studies	Generalized anxiety, GAD	While emerging data is encouraging, further placebo-controlled studies are needed. May be challenging to source from South America
Skullcap (*Scutellaria officinalis*)	Dried herb 1–2 g per day (no establizhed standardization markers)	A range of constituents, including phenolics	Minor research and traditional use detailing potential use as an anxiolytic	No adverse reactions found in studies	Generalised anxiety and stress, nervous and physical tension	May have an adjunctive role in presentations of muscular tension. More research needed
Valerian (*Valeriana* spp.)	Dried herb 1–3 g per day standardized to valepotriates and/ or valerenic acid	Valepotriates and valerenic acid	Minor research. Not strongly supportive of anxiolytic effects. Hypnotic (sleep) effects also mixed evidence for insomnia	May cause excitation, stimulation, and vivid dreams	Generalised anxiety, physical tension, insomnia	May have an adjunctive role in presentations of insomnia and/or muscular tension. May however cause excitation in some individuals. Taste and scent may be unpleasant for some

relaxant [16], anti-thrombotic [17], neuroprotective [14], mild anaesthetic [18], hypnotic [19], and anticonvulsant [14]. As briefly detailed in Table 2.1, numerous in vivo and in vitro studies from animals and humans suggest possible mechanisms, which may mediate the actions of kava extract and specific kavalactones including: blockade of voltage-gated sodium ion channels, reduced excitatory neurotransmitter release due to blockade of calcium ion channels, enhanced ligand binding to GABA type A receptors, reversible inhibition of monoamine oxidase B, and reduced neuronal re-uptake of noradrenaline (norepinephrine) and dopamine [5]. Unlike benzodiazepines, kavalactones do not bind directly to GABA receptors, and appear to achieve GABAergic effects via modulation of the GABA channels, increased binding to and upregulation of GABA binding sites [14, 20]. Davies and colleagues [21] found no significant interactions between GABA or benzodiazepine binding sites and the pharmacological activities of kava within rodents; and Boonen and Häberlein [22] discovered that kavalactones dihydromethysticin, dihydrokavain, methysticin and kavain also did not bind with GABA-α receptors in an animal model (and did not antagonise flunitrazepam binding to benzodiazepine sites).

2.2.3 Evidence of Efficacy

2.2.3.1 Anxiety

A Cochrane review has been undertaken of 11 RCTs of rigorous methodology using kava monopreparations (60–280 mg of kavalactones) in anxiety [7]. Results revealed significant anxiolytic activity of kava compared with placebo in all but one trial. A meta-analysis of seven placebo-controlled trials using the Hamilton Anxiety Scale (HAMA) found significant reductions in anxiety, with a strong clinical effect. Moderate heterogeneity was reported in respect to the type of extract used (acetone, ethanol, and type of standardization), dosage used (60–280 mg kavalactones), and the sample treated (preoperative anxiety, climacteric anxiety, state–trait or GAD diagnoses). The methodological quality of the trials was generally sound, with four of the seven trials having the maximum Jadad score of five. Similar findings were also demonstrated in another meta-analysis by Witte and colleagues [23], that included six placebo-controlled, randomized trials utilizing a standardized kava extract WS1490 in non-psychotic anxiety disorders (assessed via HAMA).

In response to safety concerns, the WHO commissioned a report in 2007 assessing the risk of kava products [24]. Recommendation 2.1.3 suggested that products from water-based suspensions should be studied and used preferentially over acetone and ethanol extracts. This approach is supported theoretically by evidence of safety from traditional use, and aqueous extracts being rich in hepatoprotective glutathione [25]. Due to this, recent research has been conducted following these guidelines. In 2009, the Kava Anxiety Depression Spectrum Study (KADSS) was published; a 3-week placebo-controlled, double-blind, crossover trial that recruited 60 adult participants with 1 month or more of elevated generalized anxiety [26]. The results revealed aqueous extract of kava (standardised to 250 mg of kavalactones per day) significantly ($p < 0.001$) reduced anxiety and depression levels on HAMA with a very large effect size (Cohen's *d*), $d = 2.24$. The aqueous extract was found to be safe and well-tolerated and importantly displayed no serious adverse effects, and no clinical liver toxicity. The qualitative research component of the study revealed that the key themes of kava consumption were a reduction in anxiety and stress, and calming or relaxing mental effects [27]. Other themes related to improvement in sleep and in somatic anxiety symptoms. Kava use did not cause any serious adverse reactions, although a few respondents reported nausea or other gastrointestinal side effects.

After KADSS, a follow-up, double-blind placebo controlled trial in 75 participants with GAD (DSM-IV diagnosed) in the absence of mood disorders, administered kava (120/240 mg of kavalactones/day depending on response) over a 6-week period [28]. Intention-to-treat (ITT) analysis was performed on 58 participants who met inclusion criteria after an initial 1-week placebo run-in phase. A significant treatment effect of moderate effect size was found for kava ($p = 0.046$, Cohen's $d = 0.62$). Among participants with moderate to severe diagnosed GAD (assessed by the MINI Plus) this effect was larger ($p = 0.02$; $d = 0.82$). Within the kava group GABA transporter polymorphisms rs2601126 ($p = 0.046$) and rs2697153 ($p = 0.02$) were associated with greater HAMA reduction. Kava also demonstrated equivalent efficacy to synthetic agents buspirone and opipramol in an 8-week 3-arm clinical trial ($n = 129$) for the treatment of ICD-10 diagnosed GAD [29]. This demonstration of equivocal efficacy is noteworthy (although the lack of a placebo arm limits a firm conclusion) as kava may provide an advantage over synthetic comparators such as benzodiazepines, in respect to limiting daytime sedation and cognitive impairment [30]. Preferential use of kava may have less potential for addiction, and be associated with less withdrawal and rebound problems compared to chronic benzodiazepine use.

2.2.3.2 Mental Function

Acute ($n = 9$) and chronic ($n = 3$) cognitive effects of kava have been measured across 12 clinical trials. All trials adopted cognitive measures, which similarly assessed visual attention, memory retrieval, and psychomotor function. Four out of ten studies suggested improved accuracy and performance on visual attention and working memory measures [31–34], while 5 out of 11 studies found kava to have little or no negative effect on cognitive processes [35–40]. One study reported kava to impair reaction time [41]. Therefore, the current evidence suggests that kava has a positive or benign effect on cognition, while impairing motor skills at higher doses. Acute RCTs that have suggested that kava significantly enhances cognitive performance attribute these effects to specific short-term physiological processes. For example, Thompson and colleagues [31] found kava improved performance in the Sperling partial report, and recognition tasks, improving the ability of selective attention, visual processing speed and the efficiency of memory retrieval [31]. The authors speculated that kava may decrease the rate of decay for images held in iconic memory, while increasing the time taken for items to be transferred to a more permanent memory trace. Response accuracy was also increased, indicating that kava may have beneficial effects on working memory and retrieval processes. This study, however, found that reaction time was reduced by 40 % in comparison to placebo, suggesting a possible negative effect on motor-skill-based tasks such as driving.

The ability of kava to inhibit the re-uptake of noradrenaline is a novel pharmacological mechanism which may differentiate it from synthetic anxiolytics (e.g. benzodiazepine) [34]. A 2012 Australian RCT [40] compared the acute neurocognitive, anxiolytic, and thymoleptic effects of a medicinal dose of kava to a benzodiazepine, and explored for the first time specific genetic polymorphisms, which may affect psychotropic activity. Twenty-two moderately anxious adults aged 18–65 years were randomized to receive an acute dose of kava (180 mg of kavalactones), oxazepam (30 mg), or placebo 1 week apart in a crossover trial. Kava and oxazepam were not found to impair cognitive performance on a computerised battery of six tests: Simple Reaction Time, Digit Vigilance Task, Choice Reaction Time, Numeric Working Memory, Rapid Visual Information Processing, and Corsi Blocks. As mentioned above, psychophysiological effects of kava vary according to a range of factors that include: the specific cultivar (extract), the dose, the method of preparation, and the person's genetics and biochemistry (in addition to potential dispositional differences).

2.3 Passionflower (*Passiflora incarnata*)

2.3.1 Overview

The herbal medicine passionflower (also known as maypop) has a long history of traditional use in stress, sleep, and anxiety disorders [42, 43]. It is claimed that the medicinal properties of passionflower were first described in 1569 by a Spanish researcher in Peru [44]. Felter and Lloyd [45] state that passionflower was first introduced as a medicine to America around 1840, with the first trials of passionflower recorded in the *New Orleans Medical Journal* around that time. In their well-regarded materia medica *King's American Dispensatory* [45], Felter and Lloyd (p. 1440) describe passionflower's medicinal action as being "exerted chiefly upon the nervous system," and state that "it is specifically useful to allay *restlessness* and overcome *wakefulness,* when these are the result of exhaustion, or the nervous excitement of debility." In addition, they state "It gives sleep to those who are labouring under the effects of mental worry or from mental overwork." These traditional descriptions have informed modern research on passionflower's anxiolytic effects.

There are a number of passionflower species used traditionally; however, research has focused on *Passiflora incarnata* (unless specified otherwise below), as it has a well-documented history of traditional use, and exhibits the strongest anxiolytic effect in comparison to other species [46]. The aerial parts of the plant have been used traditionally, with the leaves being identified as having the strongest anxiolytic action [43].

2.3.2 Mechanisms of Action

Passionflower has been found to have numerous bioactive constituents, which include amino acids [47], various β-carboline alkaloids, and flavonoids [48–50]. The flavonoid chrysin is a benzodiazapine receptor ligand [51–53]; however, it appears to have a low binding affinity to this receptor; therefore, it is suggested that other mechanisms involving the $GABA_A$ receptor could better explain passionflower's anxiolytic activity [49, 50]. While the benzoflavone compound (BZF) is considered a main active anxiolytic constituent of passionflower [48], consensus in the literature has not been reached [54]. Despite this dispute, passionflower is typically standardized to BZF content, although the amount has varied when used in clinical trials from 1.01/500 mg [55] to 2.8 mg/5 ml [56]. Results from in vitro studies using passionflower whole leaf extract have also been inconsistent. GABA transaminase was preferentially inhibited in one in vitro study [3]. In contrast, another study on rats found no effect on GABA transaminase, GABA release or the benzodiazapine receptor, while the uptake of [3-H]-GABA into rat cortical synaptosomes was inhibited [57]. The exact mechanism of action remains unclear due to inconsistencies across studies regarding the preparations used, the experimental conditions, dosage, and routes of administration, which vary considerably across studies.

2.3.2.1 In Vivo Studies

A number of studies have used animal behavioural models to measure the anxiolytic effects associated with *Passiflora* spp. whole plant extracts [43, 46, 48, 51, 54, 58–66]. All included studies demonstrated anxiolytic effects, although different preparations were used, with an anxiolytic effect seen a different doses, and sedative effects observed at higher doses [64, 66]. This section will focus on *Passiflora incarnata*, as the majority of in vivo studies have investigated this species, and it is the only species to be researched in clinical trials. Dhawan and colleagues conducted a series of acute dose escalation studies in mice [43, 46, 48, 59], all of which demonstrated that a passionflower methanol extract (methanol fraction only) was associated with a statistically significant reduction in acute anxiety in mice. There was a dose-dependent decrease in anxiety with the maximum benefit observed at 125 mg/kg, which was an equivalent effect to 2 mg/kg of diazepam [46]. The highest dose of 300 mg/kg showed no anxiolytic effect [46]. Sampath and colleagues [54] demonstrated a number of fractions of passionflower hydroethanol extract to have anxiolytic effects in mice. Using three behavioural models another study demonstrated passionflower to have dose-dependent effects in mice, with anxiolytic and sedative effects occurring at 400 mg/kg, and a sedative but non-anxiolytic effect seen at 800 mg/kg [66]. Two mice studies by Grundmann and colleagues [60, 61] confirmed two different preparations of passionflower extract to have an acute dose-dependent (375 mg/kg) anxiolytic effect comparable to diazepam.

2.3.3 Evidence of Efficacy

2.3.3.1 Clinical Studies

Passiflora incarnata has demonstrated significant reductions in anxiety symptoms in three studies [42, 55, 56]. One of the studies focused on chronic anxiety, while the other two investigated acute symptoms. A 4-week double-blind RCT used two comparison groups: passionflower extract at 45 drops/day plus placebo tablet, and placebo drops plus oxazepam at 30 mg/day, in 36 outpatients with a GAD diagnosis (DSM IV) [42]. Reductions in total mean HAMA scores ($p < 0.01$) were observed in both groups, although no significant differences were found between groups at 4 weeks. The passionflower group took longer (7 days) to demonstrate a significant reduction in HAMA scores compared to the oxazepam group (4 days). No differences in the frequency of side effects were observed; although, increased impairment in job performance was noted for the oxzepam group.

Two RCTs in preoperative patients demonstrated an acute anxiolytic effect with two different preparations of passionflower [55, 56]. The first study orally administered either a tablet containing 500 mg (1.01 mg BZF) of passionflower or placebo to patients 90 min before surgery [55]. Anxiety was measured at preoperative baseline, 10, 30, 60 and 90 min following administration, and a significant reduction in anxiety was found in both groups over time. There was also a significant difference between the two groups, with passionflower demonstrating a greater reduction in anxiety over time compared to placebo. Reduced anxiety was reported from 10 min post-dose, and peaked at 30 min. The second study used an aqueous extract of passionflower standardized to 2.8 mg BZF per 5 ml of extract (700 mg/5 ml) that was administered 30 min prior to spinal anaesthesia [56]. A significant reduction in preoperative anxiety compared to placebo—as measured by the STAI-S—was found prior to spinal anaesthesia for BZF in comparison to placebo. The anxiolytic effects similarly peaked at 30 min. Neither of these acute studies reported sedative effects or reduced psychomotor function.

While these studies provide preliminary evidence of efficacy for passionflower as an anxiolytic using chronic and acute dosing, further research is required in order to establish efficacy across a range of anxiety disorders.

2.4 Chamomile (*Matricaria recutita*)

2.4.1 Overview

Chamomile (*Matricaria recutita*) is a medicinal herb with a long history of traditional use for its calming effect. Felter and Lloyd [45] describe its action as "affecting both the sensory and motor nerves"(p. 1246) being specifically indicated for "nervous irritability, with peevishness, fretfulness, discontent, and impatience" (p. 1247). The flowering tops are the plant part most commonly used for their medicinal action. Chamomile is also widely consumed as tea for a relaxing effect [67], and is used therapeutically in tablet, capsule, liquid extract, and in essential oil form.

2.4.2 Mechanisms of Action

Preclinical research on chamomile has reported a range of anxiolytic effects involving the GABA system [3, 68]; however, the exact pharmacology and number of active constituents are yet to be determined. Flavonoids contained in chamomile have been found to act on the GABA system [3, 68]. The flavone apigenin is suggested to be a benzodiazepine receptor ligand with anxiolytic activity [52, 69]; however, it has not consistently shown an interaction with the benzodiazepine receptor [50], and it is argued that its binding affinity is low [68].

One study found apigenin to have a sedative rather than anxiolytic effect, and it was concluded that the sedative effect is related to activation of the $GABA_A$ receptor [68]. The authors suggested that other constituents with benzodiazepine-like activity are involved in the sedative effect rather than apigenin. Chamomile whole plant extract was found to inhibit both glutamic acid decarboxylase and GABA transaminase; however, inhibition of glutamic acid decarboxylase was greater than that of GABA transaminase, indicating that CNS excitation could occur [3]. This suggests that other yet to be determined mechanisms are most likely involved in chamomile's anxiolytic and sedative effects.

2.4.3 Evidence of Efficacy

A number of animal behavioural studies have explored the anxiolytic effects of isolated constituents of chamomile [50, 52, 68, 69]; however, there has been no animal model using the whole plant extract to date.

2.4.3.1 Clinical Studies

A single, double-blind, dose escalation RCT investigated the effects of chamomile on symptoms of GAD. Chamomile extract standardized to 1.2 % apigenin was found to reduce anxiety symptoms in individuals ($n = 57$) with a DSM-IV diagnosis of GAD [67]. Doses ranged from 220 to 1100 mg. For participants who demonstrated a 50 % or less reduction in total HAMA scores from weeks 3 to 4, and 5 to 8, doses were increased to between three and five capsules daily. Following 8 weeks of treatment, chamomile was demonstrated to significantly reduce anxiety symptoms (mean total HAMA scores) compared to placebo (−3.17; 95 % CI: −6.26, −0.45, $p = 0.047$) [67]. Chamomile was well-tolerated with no increase in adverse events at higher doses, compared to placebo. The study provided preliminary evidence to suggest that chamomile may reduce anxiety symptoms associated with GAD; however, further research is needed to replicate these findings and determine the most effective dose.

The above study also measured the antidepressant effects of chamomile, and found a statistically significant greater reduction in depressive symptoms (mean HAMD scores) for chamomile in comparison to placebo. It is possible that the antidepressant effects occurred as a secondary effect following the reduction of anxiety symptoms, and was not directly related to an antidepressant effect of chamomile.

Further research on chamomile should be considered in the treatment of GAD with co-morbid depression. In regard to the use of chamomile in other anxiety disorders, preliminary research is yet to be conducted.

2.5 Galphimia (*Galphimia glauca*)

2.5.1 Overview

The use of galphimia (*Galphimia glauca*) as a medicinal plant is reported to date back to the sixteenth century [70]. It is a plant medicine indigenous to Mexico, with the leaves and stem traditionally used in the treatment of a range of ailments including asthma, allergies, and nervous disorders. It is specifically indicated for treating "nervous excitement" and is considered a sedative in Mexican folk medicine [70]. Galphimia is the most widely studied herbal treatment for anxiety in Mexico.

2.5.2 Mechanisms of Action

Galphimines have been identified as active compounds in galphimia, with the nor-secotriterpenes galphimine A and galphimine B, being shown to have the strongest anxiolytic activity [71]. Galphimine B has been considered the primary active constituent for galphimia's anxiolytic and sedative effect, and is the constituent standardized for clinical trials. Galphimine B has been shown to interact with serotonergic transmission in the dorsal hippocampus in rats. This occurs by increasing the frequency of neuronal discharge in CA1 cells, resulting in activation of 5HT(1A) receptors [72]. One study in mice demonstrated that galphimines cross the blood–brain barrier, with galphimine A found to have an effect on the central nervous system [71].

2.5.3 Evidence of Efficacy

2.5.3.1 Preclinical

A number of galphimine constituents, including galphimine B, were evaluated for their anxiolytic effects in mice using the EPM [73]. Mice were intraperitoneally administered 15 mg/kg of a galaphimine derivative 1 hour before testing. An anxiolytic-like effect in the mice was found for both galphimine A and galphimine B, with a significant increase in the time spent in and number of entries into the open arm in the EPM. A second study on mice used a methanolic extract (standardized for galphimine B, 8.3 mg/g) at different doses (125, 250, 500, 1000 and 2000 mg/kg), which were orally administered at three different times (24, 18 and 1 hour before the test). Significant anxiolytic-like effects were found in the light–dark paradigm test and the EPM, but not the forced swimming test [73].

2.5.3.2 Clinical

Two clinical trials have found galphimia to be an effective anxiolytic. The first was a 4-week, positive-controlled double-blind RCT, with a cohort of 152 patients with a DSM-IV diagnosis of GAD and HAMA scores ≥19 [74]. The two groups received either galphimia aqueous extract (310 mg standardized to 0.348 mg of galphimine B), or the benzodiazepine lorazepam (1 mg). Each treatment was administered in capsule form (identical in appearance) twice daily. Both groups demonstrated a significant reduction in anxiety symptoms. There were no significant side effects reported in the galphimia group, which contrasted with the lorazepam group, in which over 21 % of people reported excessive sedation.

A second RCT investigated the effects of galphimia extract over 15 weeks on patients (n = 191) with a GAD diagnosis (DSM-IV) and HAMA scores ≥20 [75]. The galphimia group were administered two to four capsules (3.48 mg galphimia extract standardized to 0.175 mg of galphimine B) at the physician's discretion over 12 weeks, followed by 3 weeks of withdrawal. The second group received 0.5 mg of lorazepam.The galphimia treatment group had a reduction in HAMA scores that was significantly greater than the lorazepam group, with no difference between groups in tolerability of treatments.

2.6 Skullcap (*Scutellaria lateriflora*)

2.6.1 Overview

The aerial parts of skullcap (*Scutellaria lateriflora*) have been used in European and North American traditional medicine [76, 77] for anticonvulsant, relaxant, and nervous system tonic effects [78]. Research has identified diterpenoids, amino acids (GABA and glutamine), essential oil, and phenolic compounds in skullcap [78, 79]. A total of 73 bioactive constituents have been identified in the volatile oil, which include mainly sesquiterpenes [80]. Flavones appear to be the main constituents with anxiolytic actions, which include baicalein, baicalin, and wogonin [81, 82].

2.6.2 Mechanisms of Action

Flavone glycosides have been demonstrated to bind to a 5-HT_7 receptor [78]. The flavone wogonin has been found to interact with benzodiazapine receptors in the GABA system to exert an anxiolytic effect [81]. Baicalein has been identified as a benzodiazepine receptor ligand (with weak binding affinity), and demonstrated both sedative and anxiolytic effects that are mediated via GABA(A) non-benzodiazepine sites [82]. Baicalin (a metabolite of baicalein) has demonstrated selective partial GABA(A) receptor antagonism [82]. A whole plant extract (ethanol) of skullcap demonstrated anxiolytic effect via inhibition of both glutamic acid decarboxylase and GABA-transaminase, with preferential inhibition of GABA-transaminase [3].

2.7 Evidence of Efficacy

2.7.1 Preclinical

Awad and colleagues [47] administered an acute oral dose of 100 mg of skullcap aqueous extract to rats using the EPM. Results revealed that treated rats spent more time in the open arms compared to placebo, and displayed less risk assessment behaviour in the open field test. The authors identified and quantified that the flavonoids baicalin and its aglycone baicalein, as well as the amino acids GABA and glutamine, may play a role in the plant's anxiolytic activity.

2.7.2 Clinical

Two clinical trials have investigated the anxiolytic effects of skullcap. One crossover RCT investigated the anxiolytic effects of the plant medicine in healthy adults ($n = 19$) [76]. Four treatments were given to each participant: two placebo capsules, one skullcap capsule (350 mg freeze-dried), one skullcap capsule (100 mg freeze-dried extract), and two skullcap capsules (100 mg freeze-dried extract). Each treatment was of 2 hours duration, and taken at least 2 days apart. Anxiety was measured at baseline, and 30, 60, 90 and 120 min on the Acute Psycho-Activity Self-Rating Scale that indicated whether the effect was stimulating or sedating. All three skullcap treatments demonstrated anxiolytic effects, with the two 100 mg/kg skullcap capsules demonstrating the greatest effect compared to placebo. However, this study was methodologically flawed and did not report statistical data; therefore, conclusions about anxiolytic effects cannot be made.

Another crossover RCT investigated the effects of *Scutellaria lateriflora* on anxiety and mood in healthy adults ($n = 43$) [83]. Two groups received either skullcap (350 mg capsules) or placebo (*Utica dioica folia*, 300 mg capsules) for 14 days, followed by a 7-day washout period after which they took the alternative treatment for 14 days. Those assigned to the first group (P-S) had significantly higher mean anxiety scores as measured by the Beck Anxiety Inventory. Results revealed a significant difference between treatments for the first group (P-S), but not for the second group (S-P), a result that may be explained by the higher levels of anxiety in group 1. In addition, no differences in mood were found between groups, although an enhanced mood effect for skullcap was reported in group 1 (P-S), and for placebo in group 2 (S-P), which the authors suggest may be related to continued effect of skullcap following washout. It was concluded that skullcap may reduce depression symptoms in some people, although further research is warranted.

2.8 Valerian (*Valeriana* spp.)

2.8.1 Overview

The *Valeriana* spp. comprises over 200 species worldwide, with extracts from the roots having a long history of traditional use across Europe and the Americas as an antispasmodic, and more recently as a sedative [84]. The sesquiterpenoids (valerenic acid) and valepotriates are the main active constituents of valerian [85].

2.8.1.1 Mechanisms of Action

Valerian extract, in particular valerenic acid, has been found to activate adenosine receptors and potentiate synaptic GABAergic transmission via GABA(A) receptors [86, 87]. In vivo, valerenic acid has demonstrated strong anxiolytic activity in mice, using both the EPM and the light/dark choice test at 10 and 3 mg/kg p.o. [87]. There is also evidence to suggest that valepotriates potentiate GABAergic transmission [88].

2.8.2 Evidence of Efficacy

2.8.3 Preclinical

The anxiolytic action of valerian has been investigated in two animal behavioural studies. In one study, five different extraction techniques (total valerenic acids between 0.13 and 0.38 %) were used, and administered at different doses [89]. Three extracts showed a reduction in anxiety-like behaviours that were significant at doses of 100, 250 and 500 mg/kg. The strongest anxiolytic effects were demonstrated with the 35 % ethanol extract (0.29 % valerenic acids) at 100 and 250 mg/kg. In contrast with the reputed activity of valerian, none of the extracts demonstrated a sedative effect. Another study in rats demonstrated valerian extract to have a significant reduction in anxiety compared to control, which was similar to diazepam [90]. These studies indicate that further investigation is warranted with regard to the most effective extraction type and dosage regimes required for anxiolytic effects.

2.8.3.1 Clinical

One study has explored the anxiolytic effect of isolated valepotriates in chronic anxiety. This was a three-arm, double-blind, parallel-group design over 4 weeks [91]. Patients ($n = 36$) with a GAD diagnosis (DSM-III-R) received either 81.3 mg valepotriates or 6.5 mg diazepam (mean daily dose for both treatments), or placebo. Post-treatment there were no significant differences from baseline as measured by the HAMA and the STAI-Trait; however, post-treatment scores on the STAI-Trait were significantly lower in the diazepam group compared to the valerian group. As isolated valepotriates were used in this study, it is difficult to extrapolate the findings to the use of whole galenic extracts that are more commonly used. In addition, valepotriates have a cytotoxic potential and is a safety concern [92, 93], which contrasts with commercially available valerian extracts that are higher in valerenic acid [84].

An open-label study explored the effects of *Valeriana wallichii* (a species commonly used in India) on 33 adults with anxiety-stress disorder diagnosed with clinical interview [94]. Anxiety was assessed with the Brief Psychiatric Rating Scale.

Participants were given 500 mg capsules twice daily for 60 days, and a significant reduction in anxiety symptoms was found at both 30 and 60 days of treatment. As this was a small sample and there was no placebo group, it is difficult to draw strong conclusions from the results of this study.

The acute anxiolytic effects of *Valeriana officinalis* were investigated in an RCT of 20 dental patients prior to surgical removal of impacted molars [95]. Two groups received either valerian (100 mg) or placebo capsules that were identical in appearance. Physiological measures (i.e. heart rate, systolic blood pressure, diastolic blood pressure, paleness, agitation) as observed by both a researcher and surgeon were used to assess levels of anxiety. Both the observers determined a reduction in anxiety symptoms in those receiving valerian compared to placebo; however, the surgeon's assessment did not reach statistical significance. Both groups reported muscle relaxation and sleepiness, although these effects may have been caused by the surgical procedure.

2.8.4 Clinical Considerations

The herbal medicines presented in this chapter have primarily demonstrated evidence in treating diagnosed GAD and generalized anxiety symptoms. Specifically, kava, passionflower, chamomile, galphimia have demonstrated various levels of efficacy in treating anxiety symptoms associated with GAD, suggesting that they may be suitable for more chronic forms of anxiety. *Valeriana wallichii* demonstrated a reduction in anxiety symptoms over a 2-month period; however, more methodologically rigorous studies are needed to replicate this finding. The secondary sedative actions of these herbs make them particularly useful in treating anxiety presenting with sleep disturbances. In terms of more acute effects, reduction of anxiety has been demonstrated in kava, passionflower and *Valeriana officinalis* in various contexts. Kava, chamomile and skullcap have shown both anxiolytic and antidepressant effects associated with anxiety, so are worth considering in cases of co-morbid depression. Theoretically, the herbs covered in this chapter could be useful in treating other specific anxiety disorders; however, more research is needed.

Prescriptive advice for clinicians regarding the use of herbal medicines to treat anxiety involves many potential considerations. First, as in the case of all herbal medicine products, quality is an important issue as this potentially affects efficacy and safety [96]. For example, in the case of kava, current evidence suggests previous use of cheaper kava plant parts and cultivars may have been implicated in hepatotoxicity; therefore, using traditional water-soluble rhizome extracts of a noble cultivar of the plant is advised [97]. The use of traditional aqueous extracts of kava from a peeled rhizome from a "noble" chemotype (e.g. Borogu, used for its pleasant effects with the least occurrence of side effects) appears to be advisable.

The alacrity of effect of these herbal medicines appears to vary. The anxiolytic action of herbal medicines such as kava and passionflower have a rapid onset, thus may be more applicable in intermittent use when acute anxiolysis is required. Due to kava having some similarities in clinical profile to benzodiazepines—in respect to speed of onset (without the neurocognitive effects)—monitoring for abuse is advised. It should be noted that addiction to medicinal doses of kava has not been revealed [98]. Passionflower and valerian have also demonstrated acute anxiolytic effects to varying degrees in preoperative conditions; however, more research is needed to determine their usefulness in other acute forms of anxiety, and clinical disorders such as panic and social anxiety. In the cases of the other herbal medicines discussed above, it is unknown whether repeated effects are required for an anxiolytic effect to occur, or whether acute effects are evident.

Passionflower is worthy of further investigation as an anxiolytic treatment, with its traditional indication for "worry" being well-suited to those with GAD. Although passionflower has been shown to have less negative cognitive effects than benzodiazepines in both animal and human studies, more evidence is needed for efficacy and safety of longer-term treatment, as long-term treatment is often needed in those with more chronic forms of anxiety.

Apart from kava, all the discussed herbal medicines are considered to have adequate safety profiles. In terms of kava, a consideration for long-term use (or in cases of potential liver dysfunction) is to recommend routine liver function tests and hepatobiliary clinical examination. Finally, co-administration with these herbal medicines with alcohol or benzodiazepines should be approached cautiously (especially with kava), and caution should apply if the patient is taking any medications. As there is the possibility of potentiating the effects of benzodiazepines, SSRIs or depressants such as alcohol, adjunctive use of these herbal anxiolytics needs to be considered with caution. However, there is the potential for the use of these herbal anxiolytics as an adjunctive to reduce the dosage or frequency of use of benzodiazepines or SSRIs. While caution is advised in the co-use as we do not fully understand the potential interactions, research has indicated a potential application for kava in people withdrawing from benzodiazepines [99].

While pharmaceutical and herbal medicines target physiological mechanisms involved in anxiety and sleep problems, they do not directly address important psychological factors involved. For example, excessive uncontrollable worry is a defining feature of GAD, which is also involved in insomnia [100]. This symptom is usually addressed with psychological therapies (such as cognitive behavioural therapy [CBT]) focusing on dysfunctional cognitions and consequent behaviours [101]. While CBT has been found to be an effective treatment in anxiety disorders [101], there are many people who do not respond to treatment (between 34 and 36 % [102]); therefore, pharmaceuticals such as benzodiazepines are often used as adjunct treatments. As benzodiazepines have the potential for addiction and unwanted side effects, herbal anxiolytics may provide a safer, better-tolerated alternative as adjuncts to psychological therapies. In the case of treating anxiety co-morbid with insomnia, anxiolytic herbal medicines with sedative properties may be of benefit if taken in the evening as a hypnotic agent.

In summary, for all the herbal anxiolytics discussed in this chapter there is a need for future research to determine the most effective dose, extraction type, and standardisation to ensure phytoequivalence of these medicines. In addition, future research is needed to determine the effectiveness of these medicines as adjunct treatments with both pharmaceutical and psychological treatments. However, despite these limitations there is an increasing body of evidence that supports the use of these herbal medicines as an effective treatment for anxiety symptoms, especially related to GAD.

References

1. American Psychiatric Association. Diagnostic and statistical manual of mental disorders. 5th ed. Arlington: American Psychiatric Association; 2013.
2. Lebot V, Lévesque J. The origin and distribution of kava (Piper methysticum Forst. f. and Piper wichmannii C. DC., Piperaceae): a phytochemical approach. Allertonia. 1989;5:223–80.
3. Awad R et al. Effects of traditionally used anxiolytic botanicals on enzymes of the γ-aminobutyric acid (GABA) system. Can J Physiol Pharmacol. 2007;85(9):933–42.
4. Bilia AR, Gallon S, Vincieri FF. Kava-kava and anxiety: growing knowledge about the efficacy and safety. Life Sci. 2002;70(22):2581–97.
5. LaPorte E et al. Neurocognitive effects of kava (Piper methysticum): a systematic review. Hum Psychopharmacol. 2011;26(2):102–11.
6. Rickels K, Rynn M. Pharmacotherapy of generalized anxiety disorder. J Clin Psychiatry. 2002;63(Suppl 14):9–16.
7. Pittler MH, Ernst E. Kava extract for treating anxiety. Cochrane Database Syst Rev. 2003;1:CD003383.
8. Clouatre DL. Kava kava: examining new reports of toxicity. Toxicol Lett. 2004;150(1):85–96.
9. Teschke R, Schwarzenboeck A, Akinci A. Kava hepatotoxicity: a European view. N Z Med J. 2008;121(1283):90–8.
10. Raduege KM et al. Anesthetic considerations of the herbal, kava. J Clin Anesth. 2004;16(4):305–11.
11. Singh YN, Singh NN. Therapeutic potential of kava in the treatment of anxiety disorders. CNS Drugs. 2002;16(11):731–43.
12. Nerurkar PV, Dragull K, Tang CS. In vitro toxicity of kava alkaloid, pipermethystine, in HepG2 cells compared to kavalactones. Toxicol Sci. 2004;79(1):106–11.
13. Kinzler E, Kromer J, Lehmann E. Effect of a special kava extract in patients with anxiety-, tension-, and excitation states of non-psychotic genesis. Double blind study with placebos over 4 weeks. Arzneimittelforschung. 1991;41(6):584–8.
14. Gleitz J et al. The protective action of tetrodotoxin and (+/−)-kavain on anaerobic glycolysis, ATP content and intracellular Na + and Ca2+ of anoxic brain vesicles. Neuropharmacology. 1996;35(12):1743–52.
15. Jamieson DD, Duffield PH. The antinociceptive actions of kava components in mice. Clin Exp Pharmacol Physiol. 1990;17(7):495–507.
16. Singh YN. Effects of kava on neuromuscular transmission and muscle contractility. J Ethnopharmacol. 1983;7(3):267–76.
17. Gleitz J et al. Antithrombotic action of the kava pyrone (+)-kavain prepared from Piper methysticum on human platelets. Planta Med. 1997;63(1):27–30.
18. Singh HK, Dhawan BN. Neuropsychopharmacological effects of the ayurvedic nootropic Bacopa monniera Linn. (Brahmi). Indian J Pharm. 1997;29(5):S359–65.
19. Wheatley D. Stress-induced insomnia treated with kava and valerian: singly and in combination. Hum Psychopharmacol. 2001;16(4):353–6.
20. Jussofie A, Schmiz A, Hiemke C. Kavapyrone enriched extract from Piper methysticum as modulator of the GABA binding site in different regions of rat brain. Psychopharmacology (Berl). 1994;116:469–74.

21. Davies LP et al. Kava pyrones and resin: studies on GABAA, GABAB and benzodiazepine binding sites in rodent brain. Pharmacol Toxicol. 1992;71(2):120–6.
22. Boonen G, Häberlein H. Influence of genuine kavapyrone enantiomers on the GABAA binding site. Planta Med. 1998;64:504–6.
23. Witte S, Loew D, Gaus W. Meta-analysis of the efficacy of the acetonic kava-kava extract WS1490 in patients with non-psychotic anxiety disorders. Phytother Res. 2005;19(3):183–8.
24. CoulterD.Assessment of the risk of hepatotoxicity with kava products.WHO Appointed Committee.2007.
25. Whitton PA et al. Kava lactones and the kava-kava controversy. Phytochemistry. 2003;64(3):673–9.
26. Sarris J et al. The Kava Anxiety Depression Spectrum Study (KADSS): a randomized, placebo-controlled, cross-over trial using an aqueous extract of Piper methysticum. Psychopharmacology (Berl). 2009;205(3):399–407.
27. Sarris J, Adams J, Kavanagh D. An explorative qualitative analysis of participants' experience of using kava versus placebo in an RCT. Aust J Med Med Herbalism. 2010;22(1):12–6.
28. Sarris J et al. Kava in the treatment of generalized anxiety disorder: a double-blind, randomized, placebo-controlled study. J Clin Psychopharmacol. 2013;33(5):643–8.
29. Boerner RJ et al. Kava-Kava extract LI 150 is as effective as Opipramol and Buspirone in Generalised Anxiety Disorder–an 8-week randomized, double-blind multi-centre clinical trial in 129 out-patients. Phytomedicine. 2003;10(Suppl 4):38–49.
30. Buffett-Jerrott SE, Stewart SH. Cognitive and sedative effects of benzodiazepine use. Curr Pharm Des. 2002;8(1):45–58.
31. Thompson R, Ruch W, Hasenohrl RU. Enhanced cognitive performance and cheerful mood by standardized extracts of Piper methysticum (Kava-kava). Hum Psychopharmacol. 2004;19(4):243–50.
32. Saletu B et al. EEG-brain mapping, psychometric and psychophysiological studies on central effects of kavain – a kava plant derivative. Hum Psychopharmacol. 1989;4:169–90.
33. Heinze HJ et al. Pharmacopsychological effects of oxazepam and kava-extract in a visual search paradigm assessed with event-related potentials. Pharmacopsychiatry. 1994;27(6):224–30.
34. Munte TF et al. Effects of oxazepam and an extract of kava roots (Piper methysticum) on event-related potentials in a word recognition task. Neuropsychobiology. 1993;27(1):46–53.
35. Foo H, Lemon J. Acute effects of kava, alone or in combination with alcohol, on subjective measures of impairment and intoxication and on cognitive performance. Drug Alcohol Rev. 1997;16(2):147–55.
36. Prescott J et al. Acute effects of kava on measures of cognitive performance, physiological function and mood. Drug Alcohol Rev. 1993;12(1):49–57.
37. Russell PN, Bakker D, Singh NN. The effects of kava on altering and speed of access of information from long-term memory. Bull Psychon Soc. 1987;25(4):236–7.
38. Mathews JD et al. Effects of the heavy usage of kava on physical health: summary of a pilot survey in an aboriginal community. Med J Aust. 1988;148(11):548–55.
39. CairneySetal.Saccadeandcognitivefunctioninchronickavausers.Neuropsychopharmacology. 2003;28(2):389–96.
40. Sarris J et al. The acute effects of kava and oxazepam on anxiety, mood, neurocognition; and genetic correlates: a randomized, placebo-controlled, double-blind study. Hum Psychopharmacol. 2012;27(3):262–9.
41. Cairney S et al. Saccade and cognitive impairment associated with kava intoxication. Hum Psychopharmacol. 2003;18(7):525–33.
42. Akhondzadeh S et al. Passionflower in the treatment of generalized anxiety: a pilot double-blind randomized controlled trial with oxazepam. J Clin Pharm Ther. 2001;26(5):363–7.

43. Dhawan K, Kumar S, Sharma A. Anxiolytic activity of aerial and underground parts of Passiflora incarnata. J Ethnopharmacol. 2001;72(8):922–6.
44. Dhawan K, Dhawan S, Sharma A. Passiflora: a review update. J Ethnopharmacol. 2004;94(1):1–23.
45. Felter HW, Lloyd JU. King's American dispensatory. 1898.
46. Dhawan K, Kumar S, Sharma A. Comparative biological activity study on Passiflora incarnata and P. edulis. Fitoterapia. 2001;72(6):698–702.
47. Awad R et al. Phytochemical and biological analysis of skullcap (Scutellaria lateriflora L.): a medicinal plant with anxiolytic properties. Phytomedicine. 2003;10(8):640–9.
48. Dhawan K, Kumar S, Sharma A. Anti-anxiety studies on extracts of Passiflora incarnata Linneaus. J Ethnopharmacol. 2001;78(2–3):165–70.
49. Brown E et al. Evaluation of the anxiolytic effects of chrysin, a Passiflora incarnata extract, in the laboratory rat. AANA J. 2007;75(5):333–7.
50. Zanoli P, Avallone R, Baraldi M. Behavioral characterisation of the flavonoids apigenin and chrysin. Fitoterapia. 2000;71(Suppl 1):S117–23.
51. de Castro PCF et al. Possible anxiolytic effect of two extracts of Passiflora quadrangularis L. in experimental models. Phytother Res. 2007;21(5):481–4.
52. Salgueiro JB et al. Anxiolytic natural and synthetic flavonoid ligands of the central benzodiazepine receptor have no effect on memory tasks in rats. Pharmacol Biochem Behav. 1997;58(4):887–91.
53. Wolfman C et al. Possible anxiolytic effects of chrysin, a central benzodiazepine receptor ligand isolated from Passiflora Coerulea. Pharmacol Biochem Behav. 1994;47(1):1–4.
54. Sampath C et al. Anxiolytic effects of fractions obtained from Passiflora incarnata L. in the elevated plus maze in mice. Phytother Res. 2011;25(6):789–95.
55. Movafegh A et al. Preoperative oral Passiflora incarnata reduces anxiety in ambulatory surgery patients: a double-blind, placebo-controlled study. Anesth Analg. 2008;106(6):1728–32.
56. Aslanargun P et al. Passiflora incarnata Linneaus as an anxiolytic before spinal anesthesia. J Anesth. 2012;26(1):39–44.
57. Appel K et al. Modulation of the γ-aminobutyric acid (GABA) system by Passiflora incarnata L. Phytother Res. 2011;25(6):838–43.
58. Petry RD et al. Comparative pharmacological study of hydroethanol extracts of Passiflora alata and Passiflora edulis leaves. Phytother Res. 2001;15(2):162–4.
59. Dhawan K, Kumar S, Sharma A. Comparative anxiolytic activity profile of various preparations of Passiflora incarnata linneaus: a comment on medicinal plants' standardization. J Altern Complement Med. 2002;8(3):283–91.
60. Grundmann O et al. Anxiolytic effects of a passion flower (Passiflora incarnata L.) extract in the elevated plus maze in mice. Die Pharmazie(An International Journal of Pharmaceutical Sciences). 2009;64(1):63–4.
61. Grundmann O et al. Anxiolytic activity of a phytochemically characterized Passiflora incarnata extract is mediated via the GABAergic system. Planta Med. 2008;74(15):1769–73.
62. Barbosa PR et al. The aqueous extracts of Passiflora alata and Passiflora edulis reduce anxiety-related behaviors without affecting memory process in rats. J Med Food. 2008;11(2):282–8.
63. Deng J et al. Anxiolytic and sedative activities of Passiflora edulis f. flavicarpa. J Ethnopharmacol. 2010;128(1):148–53.
64. Li H et al. Comparative studies on anxiolytic activities and flavonoid compositions of Passiflora edulis 'edulis' and Passiflora edulis 'flavicarpa'. J Ethnopharmacol. 2011;133(3):1085–90.
65. Lolli LF et al. Possible involvement of GABAA-benzodiazepine receptor in the anxiolytic-like effect induced by Passiflora actinia extracts in mice. J Ethnopharmacol. 2007;111(2):308–14.

66. Soulimani R et al. Behavioural effects of Passiflora incarnata L. and its indole alkaloid and flavonoid derivatives and maltol in the mouse. J Ethnopharmacol. 1997;57(1): 11–20.
67. Amsterdam JD et al. A randomized, double-blind, placebo-controlled trial of oral Matricaria recutita (chamomile) extract therapy for generalized anxiety disorder. J Clin Psychopharmacol. 2009;29(4):378–82. doi:10.1097/JCP.0b013e3181ac935c.
68. Avallone R et al. Pharmacological profile of apigenin, a flavonoid isolated from Matricaria chamomilla. Biochem Pharmacol. 2000;59(11):1387–94.
69. Viola H et al. Apigenin, a component of Matricaria recutita flowers, is a central benzodiazepine receptors-ligand with anxiolytic effects. Planta Med. 1995;61(3):213–6.
70. Gutiérrez SLG, Chilpa RR, Jaime HB. Medicinal plants for the treatment of "nervios", anxiety, and depression in Mexican Traditional Medicine. Rev Bras Farmacogn. 2014;24(5):591–608.
71. Abarca Vargas R et al. Pharmacokinetic study in mice of galphimine-A, an anxiolytic compound from Galphimia glauca. Molecules. 2014;19(3):3120–34.
72. Jimenez-Ferrer E et al. Interaction of the natural anxiolytic Galphimine-B with serotonergic drugs on dorsal hippocampus in rats. J Ethnopharmacol. 2011;137(1):724–9.
73. Herrera-Ruiz M et al. Anxiolytic and antidepressant-like activity of a standardized extract from Galphimia glauca. Phytomedicine. 2006;13(1–2):23–8.
74. Herrera-Arellano A et al. Efficacy and tolerability of a standardized herbal product from Galphimia glauca on generalized anxiety disorder. A randomized, double-blind clinical trial controlled with lorazepam. Planta Med. 2007;73(8):713–7.
75. Herrera-Arellano A et al. Therapeutic effectiveness of galphimia glauca vslorazepam in generalized anxiety disorder. A controlled 15-week clinical trial. Planta Med. 2012;78(14):1529–35.
76. Wolfson P, Hoffmann D. An investigation into the efficacy of Scutellaria lateriflora in healthy volunteers. Altern Ther Health Med. 2003;9(2):74.
77. Li J et al. Identification of phenolic compounds from Scutellaria lateriflora by liquid chromatography with ultraviolet photodiode array and electrospray ionization tandem mass spectrometry. J Pharm Biomed Anal. 2012;63(0):120–7.
78. Zhang Z et al. Characterization of chemical ingredients and anticonvulsant activity of American skullcap (Scutellaria lateriflora). Phytomedicine. 2009;16(5):485–93.
79. Kuroda M, Iwabuchi K, Mimaki Y. Chemical constituents of the aerial parts of Scutellaria lateriflora and their alpha-glucosidase inhibitory activities. Nat Prod Commun. 2012;7(4):471.
80. Yaghmai MS. Volatile constituents of Scutellaria lateriflora L. Flavour Frag J. 1988;3(1):27–31.
81. Hui KM et al. Anxiolytic effect of wogonin, a benzodiazepine receptor ligand isolated from Scutellaria baicalensis Georgi. Biochem Pharmacol. 2002;64(9):1415–24.
82. de Carvalho RSM, Duarte FS, de Lima TCM. Involvement of GABAergic non-benzodiazepine sites in the anxiolytic-like and sedative effects of the flavonoid baicalein in mice. Behav Brain Res. 2011;221(1):75–82.
83. Brock C et al. American Skullcap (Scutellaria lateriflora): a randomised, double-blind placebo-controlled crossover study of its effects on mood in healthy volunteers. Phytother Res. 2014;28(5):692–8.
84. Gao XQ, Björk L. Valerenic acid derivatives and valepotriates among individuals, varieties and species of Valeriana. Fitoterapia. 2000;71(1):19–24.
85. Patočka J, Jakl J. Biomedically relevant chemical constituents of Valeriana officinalis. J Appl Biomed. 2010;8(11–18).
86. Muller CE et al. Interactions of valerian extracts and a fixed valerian-hop extract combination with adenosine receptors. Life Sci. 2002;71(16):1939–49.
87. Benke D et al. GABA(A) receptors as in vivo substrate for the anxiolytic action of valerenic acid, a major constituent of valerian root extracts. Neuropharmacology. 2009;56(1):174–81.

88. Dunayev VV et al. Biological activity of the sum of valepotriates isolated from Val. alliariifolia Adams. Farmakol Toksikol. 1987;50(6):33–7.
89. Hattesohl M et al. Extracts of Valeriana officinalis L. s.l. show anxiolytic and antidepressant effects but neither sedative nor myorelaxant properties. Phytomedicine. 2008;15(1–2):2–15.
90. Murphy K et al. Valeriana officinalis root extracts have potent anxiolytic effects in laboratory rats. Phytomedicine. 2010;17(8–9):674–8.
91. Andreatini R et al. Effect of valepotriates (valerian extract) in generalized anxiety disorder: a randomized placebo-controlled pilot study. Phytother Res. 2002;16(7):650–4.
92. Bos R et al. Cytotoxic potential of valerian constituents and valerian tinctures. Phytomedicine. 1998;5(3):219–25.
93. Bounthanh C et al. Valepotriates, a new class of cytotoxic and antitumor agents. Planta Med. 1981;41(1):21–8.
94. Bhattacharyya D et al. Initial exploratory observational pharmacology of Valeriana wallichii on stress management: a clinical report. Nepal Med CollJ(NMCJ). 2007;9(1):36–9.
95. Pinheiro ML et al. Valeriana officinalis L. for conscious sedation of patients submitted to impacted lower third molar surgery: a randomized, double-blind, placebo-controlled split-mouth study. J Pharm Bioallied Sci. 2014;6(2):109–14.
96. Sarris J. Current challenges in appraising complementary medicine evidence. Med J Aust. 2012;196(5):310–1.
97. Teschke R et al. Kava, the anxiolytic herb: back to basics to prevent liver injury? Br J Clin Pharmacol. 2011;71(3):445–8.
98. Sarris J, LaPorte E, Schweitzer I. Kava: a comprehensive review of efficacy, safety, and psychopharmacology. Aust N Z J Psychiatry. 2011;45(1):27–35.
99. Malsch U, Kieser M. Efficacy of kava-kava in the treatment of non-psychotic anxiety, following pretreatment with benzodiazepines. Psychopharmacology (Berl). 2001;157:277–83.
100. Carney CE et al. Distinguishing rumination from worry in clinical insomnia. Behav Res Ther. 2010;48(6):540–6.
101. Hanrahan F et al. A meta-analysis of cognitive therapy for worry in generalized anxiety disorder. Clin Psychol Rev. 2013;33(1):120–32.
102. Taylor S, Abramowitz JS, McKay D. Non-adherence and non-response in the treatment of anxiety disorders. J Anxiety Disord. 2012;26(5):583–9.

3 Adaptogens

Naomi L. Perry and David A. Camfield

3.1 Introduction

The stress response is the body's physiological response to physical and mental threats, and has evolved from the "fight or flight" response to physical danger. However, prolonged exposure to stress results in chronic engagement of this response and may lead to increased blood pressure, heart rate and blood sugar, as well as a variety of pathological conditions [1]. Stress refers to a challenge to a person's ability to adapt to inner and outer demands, and is induced by stressors such as work, bereavement or family issues [2]. Stress often manifests alongside anxiety and can result in a decline in overall health. Whilst benzodiazepines and other prescription drugs may be effective in the treatment of stress associated with anxiety disorders, the adverse effects they induce can negate the beneficial outcomes; therefore, alternative therapies are of great interest.

Adaptogens are medicinal plant compounds that have been found to enhance non-specific resistance to stress and facilitate optimal concentration, performance and endurance during periods of high stress [3, 4]. They are able to regulate physiologic processes and thereby stabilise the body's response to stress through acting on the hypothalamic–pituitary–adrenal (HPA) axis and the neuroendocrine system. Adaptogenic action has been described as a pharmacological effect of these

N.L. Perry (✉)
Centre for Human Psychopharmacology, Swinburne University of Technology,
427–451 Burwood Rd, Hawthorn, VIC, Australia
e-mail: naomiperry21@gmail.com

D.A. Camfield
Centre for Human Psychopharmacology, Swinburne University of Technology,
400 Burwood Rd, Hawthorn, VIC, Australia

School of Psychology, University of Wollongong, Wollongong, NSW, Australia

D. Camfield et al. (eds.), *Evidence-Based Herbal and Nutritional Treatments for Anxiety in Psychiatric Disorders*, DOI 10.1007/978-3-319-42307-4_3

compounds which is associated with increased resistance to the harmful effects of various stressors [5].

In this chapter, the findings from research on several well-known adaptogens will be presented and discussed, including Ashwagandha (*Withania somnifera*), Roseroot (*Rhodiola rosea*), Gotu Kola (*Centella asiatica*), Siberian Ginseng (*Eleutherococcus senticosus*) and Schisandra (*Schisandra chinensis*). The chapter summarises the current knowledge regarding the pharmacological activity of these adaptogens as well as their efficacy in the treatment of stress and anxiety associated with clinical disorders, and, where appropriate, recommendations will be given for the most effective and safe doses.

3.2 Ashwagandha (*Withania somnifera*)

3.2.1 Overview

Ashwagandha (*Withania somnifera; WS*) is an Ayurvedic herb of the *Solanaceae* family that has been used as a broad-spectrum remedy in India for centuries, with the roots being classified as a "rasayana," a medicine used to enhance both physical and mental performance [6]. WS has recognised anti-inflammatory [3, 7] and antioxidant properties [8] and is often referred to as "Indian Ginseng" due to its use in India in a similar way to the use of Ginseng in traditional Chinese medicine, which is to "balance life forces" during stress and ageing. It is often included in formulations for the treatment of musculoskeletal conditions and as a broad tonic to increase energy and improve general health. However, it has only recently been investigated in laboratory settings specifically for the treatment of stress and anxiety.

3.2.1.1 Mechanisms of Action

It has been reported that WS comprises over 35 chemical constituents, of which the biologically active compounds are alkaloids, steroidal lactones, saponins containing an additional acyl group, and withanolides with a glucose at carbon 27 [8]. Withaferin A and Withanolide D are thought to be important active constituents with regard to the adaptogenic effects of this plant [9, 10]. WS has been shown to possess GABA-mimetic properties [11, 12] and it is thought that these properties may underlie the anxiolytic effects of WS. Antioxidant activity of glycowithanolides may also explain the anti-stress effects of WS [6].

3.2.2 Evidence of Efficacy

3.2.2.1 Preclinical Studies

Anxiolytic effects and increased stress tolerance have been demonstrated with WS treatment in animal models such as exposure to shock [13], forced restraint [14] and cold water swimming tests [15]. In addition, physiological markers of stress, such as blood urea nitrogen levels, blood lactic acid and adrenal hypertrophy reduce with

WS treatment [16], as well as attenuation of stress-related parameters such as cortisol levels and sexual dysfunction in rats [13].

In a comparative study of WS and *Panax ginseng*, both plant extracts significantly reduced stress compared with saline control. However, WS showed superior effects on anabolic activity evidenced by weight gain in mice [17]. In addition, WS has been found to have benefits over Ginseng as it does not appear to result in "Ginseng abuse syndrome," which is characterised by high blood pressure, water retention, muscle tension and insomnia [17]. Additionally, the anxiolytic effects of WS have been found to be comparable to benzodiazepines, as anxiolytic effects in the elevated plus maze, social interactions and feeding latency in an unfamiliar environment were equal to lorazepam [18]. This indicates that WS may have similar efficacy to prescription drugs, but with a more favourable side-effect profile [18].

3.2.2.2 Clinical Studies

Whilst preclinical studies have demonstrated acute effects of WS on stress (e.g. [14]), the human trials that are available for review demonstrate only chronic effects. Whether WS is effective acutely in humans is currently unknown. A recent systematic review revealed that of the 62 WS human trials that have been conducted to date, only five studies met inclusion criteria for being randomised placebo-controlled trials (RCTs) in human subjects and also included a treatment arm with WS as a remedy for stress or anxiety [19]. These studies, along with clinical studies of other adaptogens, are presented in Table 3.1.

In an RCT in clinically anxious patients, a significantly greater proportion of patients receiving WS met the criteria for response than those in the placebo group following 6-week treatment [20]. Clinical response was defined as a reduction in Hamilton Anxiety Scale (HAM) score to below 12 and a Global Rating Scale (GRS, both patient and rater) of not more than one (ratings from 0 = no symptoms to 4 = very severe symptoms). However, the titration schedule for this study was left to the discretion of the treating physician, with doses increased up to a maximum of 2.5 g per day. For this reason it is difficult to ascertain the most effective dosage across participants using these data. However, a more recent study by Auddy and colleagues [21] addressed this issue by randomising 130 participants to receive WS 125 mg once daily, 125 mg twice daily, or 250 mg twice daily, versus placebo for 60 days. A dose-dependent improvement was observed for HAM score, suggesting that higher doses may be more effective for the treatment of anxiety.

In a third clinical study using WS, Cooley and colleagues [22] divided participants with moderate to severe anxiety of longer than 6 weeks' duration into two groups who received either weekly counselling sessions from a naturopathic doctor as well as 600 mg/day WS, or cognitive-behavioural therapy (CBT) sessions and placebo. Anxiety was significantly reduced in the naturopathic care group compared with the psychotherapy group. Whilst this study was placebo-controlled, it was not double-blinded as the care providers could not be blinded to participant distribution. The inclusion of psychotherapy techniques for one group but not the other also meant that groups were exposed to different factors besides WS treatment alone.

Table 3.1 Summary of adaptogens and their potential utility for stress and anxiety

Herbal medicine	Dosage	Major/active constituents	Key evidence	PotentialAEs	Potentialclinical use	Clinical advice
Ashwagandha (*Withania somnifera*)	Total dose of 500–1000 mg/day dried extract standardised to withanolides, or 4–6 g/day root powder	Withaferin A and Withanolide D	Mainly positive RCTs and open-label studies demonstrating efficacy as an anxiolytic and stress reducer. One RCT showing no superiority over placebo with use of a high dose, and a systematic review concluding that evidence is poor quality	Only mild adverse events reported. No interaction found with SSRIs	General anxiety; Potential use in OCD alongside SSRIs; no data on other anxiety disorders	Generally safe and well-tolerated. Appears to be safe for co-use with SSRIs. Further research needed to determine acute effects
Roseroot (*Rhodiola rosea*)	170 mg SHR-5 extract standardised to salidroside and rhodioloside for acute or chronic use. 300–600 mg/day generally recommended for chronic daily use	Salidroside, rhodioloside and rosavins	Several RCTs demonstrating anxiolytic effects and efficacy for increased working capacity in fatigued individuals when administered chronically. One review concluding that *R. rosea* is the most effective adaptogen for acute use	May have side effects such as irritability or insomnia. No interactions with drugs reported, although inhibition of proteins involved in drug metabolism have been reported	GAD; stress and fatigue; no data on other disorders. May be useful for Social Anxiety given the demonstrated acute effects	Not recommended for patients with bipolar disorder or insomnia due to potential side effects, but otherwise safe and well-tolerated. Although no interactions with drugs have been reported, if co-used with other drugs this should be carefully monitored due to the potential for increased bioavailability of these drugs

Gotu Kola (*Centella asiatica*)	Crude herb 0.5–6 g/day; Triterpenoid fraction of Centella asiatica 60–120 mg/day standardised to asiaticoside, Asiatic acid and madecassic acid	Asiaticoside	Some evidence for anxiolytic effects as well as improving cognition and quality of life, although only preliminary data are available	Mild adverse reactions reported, including skin reactions and upset stomach. Hepatotoxicity has also been reported although the dose used in these cases is not known	Possible use for GAD, although only one small, open-label study supporting this. No other clinical disorders studied	Not recommended for use in pregnant or breastfeeding women, or for longer than 6 weeks due to potential adverse reactions. Regular liver function tests may be warranted. Further large, placebo-controlled studies are needed, particularly in clinical populations
Siberian Ginseng (*Eleutherococcus senticosus*)	Dried herb 300–800 mg/day standardised to eleutherosides	Eleutherosides, triterpenoidsaponins and glycans	Numerous clinical trials demonstrating efficacy over placebo in improving mental work capacity, reducing stress and fatigue. Some evidence for superior stress-reducing effects over *Panax ginseng*	No adverse reactions reported in studies. Further research required regarding potential interactions	Chronic fatigue; stress; no data on other clinical disorders	Maximal effects achieved around 4 weeks, therefore usually administered for around 6 weeks followed by a 1–2 week break. Further research needed in clinical populations

(continued)

Table 3.1 (continued)

Herbal medicine	Dosage	Major/active constituents	Key evidence	PotentialAEs	Potentialclinical use	Clinical advice
Schisandra (*Schisandra chinensis*)	Tincture 0.5–2.0 mL; seed powder 0.25–3 g; tablets 50–200 mg standardised to schisandrin and γ-schizandrin	Chemical composition not fully known, key constituents believed to be schisandrin and gomisin	Demonstrated efficacy for increased working capacity when used acutely. Some evidence that repeated administration up to 10 days is also beneficial. One RCT showing longer treatment may result in detrimental effects	Excitability, sleeplessness and depression reported in a minority of subjects when administered daily for 2 weeks or more	Efficacy in fatigued individuals, data from clinical populations lacking	Based on reports of excitability and sleeplessness following long-term administration, intermittent use is recommended. No herb–drug interactions reported and appears to be safe for co-use with cancer drugs
ADAPT-232 (*R. rosea, S. chinensis and E. senticosus*)	Acute dose: 270 mg tablet standardised to rhodioloside, rosavin, tyrosol, schizandrin, γ-schizandrin and eleutherosides B and E	Rhodioloside, rosavin, tyrosol, schizandrin, γ-schizandrin and eleutherosides B and E	Several RCTs showing improved cognition and working capacity in stressed and fatigued individuals following acute administration. Also some evidence for efficacy in improving quality of life and reducing length of illness in pneumonia patients	No adverse reactions reported	Long-term stress, no data from clinically anxious patients at this stage	May be effective if used acutely for patients presenting with fatigue or stress. Further research needed to determine chronic effects, and whether effective for clinically diagnosed disorders such as GAD

Using 600 mg/day WS compared with placebo, Chandrasekhar and colleagues [23] reported significant improvements in scores on the Perceived Stress Scale (PSS-10) and the General Health Questionnaire (GHQ-28), as well as reductions in levels of serum cortisol using a non-clinical adult sample. Interestingly, a much higher dose of 12 g/day resulted in non-significant differences in HAM scores versus placebo [24]. Only scores for "anxious mood," an item on the HAM, showed a significant difference between groups. When taken together with the other findings mentioned above, this suggests an inverted U-shaped dose response curve regarding the effects of WS on stress and anxiety, with clarification from future studies required.

In a recent double-blind RCT, 30 patients diagnosed with Obsessive-Compulsive Disorder (OCD) according to DSM-IV criteria received either adjunctive 120 mg/day WS or placebo for 6 weeks, in addition to stable treatment on selective serotonin re-uptake inhibitors (SSRIs). A significant treatment effect was found in favour of WS, as measured by symptom severity on the Yale-Brown Obsessive-Compulsive Scale (Y-BOCS). The authors concluded that WS may be an effective adjunct to SSRIs in the treatment of OCD [25].

In addition to the RCTs detailed above, open-label studies have also shown positive effects of WS, with 2 g/day WS root powder for 3 months resulting in lowered blood pressure in subjects with stress-oriented hypertension [26]. Although the decrease in diastolic blood pressure was significant when the supplement was given with either water or milk, the decrease in systolic blood pressure only reached significance for those who took the supplement with milk. It is therefore recommended on the basis of this study that for patients with stress-related hypertension WS root powder is taken with milk.

3.2.2.3 Safety

Although, the general daily dosage WS recommendation is 500–1000 mg of an extract standardised to 1–2 % withanolides [27], doses used in human clinical trials have generally been in the range of 4–6 g/day WS root [26]. Clinical trials have reported no significant differences in adverse events compared with placebo, with the only adverse events found being mild in severity, for example, gastrointestinal upset, overstimulation and "feeling warm" [20, 22, 23]. Even doses as high as 12 g/day have been reported to be well-tolerated with no adverse reactions [24]. When administered alongside SSRIs, no adverse events have been reported either, suggesting that WS does not interact negatively with these drugs [25].

3.3 Roseroot (*Rhodiola rosea*)

3.3.1 Overview

A member of the *Crassulaceae* family, Roseroot (*Rhodiola rosea*) has long been used as a medicinal plant in Europe. *R. rosea* is grown in dry ground in the Arctic and Alpine regions of Europe, Asia and America, and whilst the green aerial part of the plant is used as a food ingredient, the root-stock is used in medicine. The use of *R. rosea* in medicine also dates back to the ancient Greeks [28], and traditional uses in countries such as England, Germany and Tibet include treatment for headache, use as a "brain tonic" and treatment of lung diseases. Roseroot has also traditionally been used as an anti-stress agent to reduce symptoms such as irritability, cognitive dysfunction and fatigue [29]. However, it is in Russia that the use of *R. rosea* as a stimulant and anti-stress treatment has been most extensive.

3.3.1.1 Mechanism of Action

The main active substance regarding the adaptogenic effects of *R. rosea* has been identified as salidroside, a phenylpropanoide derived from phenylethane [5, 30]. However, other compounds are also considered to be active adaptogenic constituents, including the phenylpropane rosavins [29, 31]. The stimulant and anti-stress actions of *R. rosea* and the glycoside salidroside have been extensively studied in Russia since they were first discovered in the 1960s [32–34]. The adaptogenic properties of *R. rosea* and salidroside have been well-documented [35–37] with the stimulant effect of these substances reported to play an important role [5, 33]. The extract SHR-5, manufactured by Swedish Herbal Institute, was characterised by HPLC-fingerprint analysis and standardised on the p-tyrosol-glucoside salidroside [30]. Olsson and colleagues [38] reported that the SHR-5 extract is standardised for rhodioloside (4 mg per 144 mg tablet) and appears to be a 70 % ethanolic extract with a 4:1 drug:extract ratio.

Evidence suggests that *R. rosea* inhibits monoamine oxidase and catechol-O-methyltransferase activity, thus modulating brain levels of monoamines, including serotonin and dopamine [39, 40]. Brain levels of these neurotransmitters may also be enhanced through increased permeability of the blood–brain barrier to their precursors [5]. Additionally, there is some evidence that *R. rosea* may affect the opioid system [41], and effects on cortisol secretion and HPA axis regulation and mediation of kinase enzymes have also been reported in the literature [29].

3.3.1.2 Preclinical Studies

Much of the research on the adaptogenic effects of *R. rosea* is unavailable for review due to its publication in Russia; however, the available literature suggests that *R. rosea* increases resistance to a wide variety of stressors: with *R. rosea* extracts found to protect against the harmful effects of oxygen, cold, radiation and heavy physical exercise as well as increasing working capacity, decreasing fatigue, improving learning and long-term memory, and regulating brain function in rodents [35, 42]. The majority of these studies investigated the effects of single-dose administration with significant acute effects seen within 1–2 h post-dose; however, Petkov and colleagues [35] demonstrated improved memory using a maze model 24 h post-dose, as well as long-term memory of this maze after 10 days' treatment.

3.3.1.3 Clinical Studies

In human studies a protective effect of *R. rosea* against the detrimental effects of stress and anxiety has similarly been demonstrated. In a review of the acute effects of adaptogens conducted by Panossian and Wagner [43] *R. rosea* was reported to be the most active of the adaptogens discussed, with evidence produced to demonstrate its stimulant effects.The standardised SHR-5 extract was used by Shevtsov and colleagues [30] in an RCT investigating the acute effects of *R. rosea* on capacity for mental work. Stressed and fatigued military cadets were administered either two (370 mg *R. rosea*) or three capsules (555 mg *R. rosea*), with both doses found to significantly reduce fatigue, as reflected in an anti-fatigue index based on performance of a variety of mental tasks. Beneficial effects on pulse pressure were also reported.

In a larger crossover RCT, Darbinyan and colleagues [5] investigated the effect of repeated low-dose *R. rosea* treatment on work-related fatigue. Fifty-six young, healthy physicians were assigned to receive 170 mg SHR-5 or placebo for 2 weeks in a crossover design, with an intermediate washout period of 2 weeks. The Fatigue Index was found to be significantly improved after 2 weeks' *R. rosea* treatment compared with placebo, suggesting that *R. rosea* can be useful in reducing fatigue in stressful work situations. However, closer examination revealed that this effect was only significant when the night duty was shorter. When participants had longer night shifts, the dose administered was not sufficient to reduce fatigue. Future studies could aim to investigate the doses necessary for effects in situations of higher levels of fatigue and stress.

In addition to the anti-fatigue effects in non-clinical samples, chronic effects of *R. rosea* have also been demonstrated in patients with Generalised Anxiety Disorder (GAD). In a small open-label study, ten GAD patients received 170 mg *R. rosea* in the form of standardised SHR-5 tablets twice daily for 10 weeks [44]. A significant reduction in anxiety following this intervention was found on the Hamilton Anxiety Rating Scale (HARS) and the anxiety subscale of the Four Dimensional Anxiety and Depression Scale. Four participants were classed as achieving remission, defined as a score of ≤8 on the HARS and a score of 1 or 2 on Clinical Global Impressions of Improvement (CGI-I). Half the sample had ≥50 % reduction in scores on the HAM-A scale, suggesting clinical as well as statistical significance. However, the lack of placebo control in this study, as well as the small sample size, makes it difficult to draw firm conclusions about the efficacy of this extract in GAD.

3.3.1.4 Safety

The most common side effects of *R. rosea* involves irritability and insomnia [44], suggesting a possible stimulating effect. It has therefore been recommended that this extract not be used in patients with bipolar disorder [45]. In addition, there may be inhibitory effects on CYP3A4 and p-glycoprotein that should be considered [46]. Inhibition of these proteins affects drug metabolism and can lead to increased bioavailability of drugs; therefore, potential interactions should be examined prior to commencing *R. rosea* supplementation. On the other hand, general daily dose recommendations are in the range of 300–600 mg, with no known interactions with other drugs or herbs [27]. Repeated administration is thought to be safe, with no adverse events reported following 2 weeks' treatment with 170 mg *R. rosea* [5].

3.4 Gotu Kola (*Centella asiatica*)

3.4.1 Overview

Gotu Kola (*Centella asiatica*) has been used traditionally in both Ayurvedic and Chinese medicine to treat anxiety and depression, and to assist meditation by producing a calming effect on the mind [47–49]. The people of Java and other Indonesian islands have also used *C. asiatica* for the treatment of other medical conditions including leprosy, eczema, diarrhoea, amenorrhea and fever [50]. The plant belongs to the *Umbellifere (Apiaceae)* family and is found throughout India up to an altitude of 1800 m, as well as in swampy areas of many tropical and subtropical countries. The whole plant is used for medicinal purposes, usually administered in the form of capsules, teas or tinctures. It contains compounds such as triterpene acids, fatty oil, glycosides and flavonoids [50].

3.4.1.1 Mechanism of Action

The main biologically active components of *C. asiatica* are saponins (also called triterpenoids), which include asiaticosides amongst others [50]. A pharmacokinetic study of total triterpenoid fraction of *Centella asiatica* (TTFCA) suggests that the active compounds are well-absorbed in humans [51]. Peak plasma levels of Asiatic acid were reached 4.5 and 4.2 h following oral administration of 30 mg and 60 mg of extract, respectively. Plasma half-lives were 2.2 h in the 30 mg dose and 3.4 h in the 60 mg dose. Saponin levels were not detectable after 24 h post-dose. Repeated treatment over 7 days resulted in higher peak plasma concentrations, longer half-lives and greater area-under-the-curve absorption values [51].

With regard to anxiolytic effects, the main constituent of *C. asiatica* is the triterpineglycoside asiaticoside, as demonstrated in both in vitro and in vivo studies [49, 52]. Triterpines in *C. asiatica* increase serotonin, noradrenaline and dopamine in the brain, as well as reduce serum corticosterone levels [52]. It is thought that this is the mechanism through which *C. asiatica* has calming effects. It has also been postulated that *C. asiatica* may exert anxiolytic effects through increased GABA activity. An ethanolic extract was shown to increase GABA levels in mice [53], whilst an aqueous extract stimulated Glutamic Acid Decarboxylase (GAD) by over 40 % at a dose of 1 mg/mL in vitro [54]. Activity at the $GABA_A$ receptor has also been demonstrated [55]. In addition, the anxiolytic activity may be in part due to binding to cholecystokinin receptors [56].

3.4.1.2 Preclinical Studies

Anti-stress and anxiolytic effects of *C. asiatica* have been demonstrated using animal models. Long-term pretreatment resulted in enhanced elevated plus maze (EPM) performance and attenuated acoustic startle response (ASR), whilst gastric ulceration induced by cold and restraint stress was significantly inhibited [53]. The isolated compound asiaticoside has also been found to have anxiolytic effects at various doses [57]. However, it has been proposed that the method by which active compounds are extracted may affect the efficacy of this plant as an anxiolytic. In one study in rats only the methanol and ethyl acetate extracts, along with isolated asiaticoside, showed anxiolytic effects when using the EPM for 5 min [49]. Importantly, asiaticoside did not affect locomotor activity, suggesting that these compounds are without sedative effects in rodents. Using a rat model to determine whether the triterpenoid Asiatic Acid (AA) had anxiolytic effects, Ceremuga and colleagues [55] found that rats treated with AA spent more time in the open arms of the EPM, although the difference was non-significant. When administered with the benzodiazepine midazolam the effect reached statistical significance, which the authors attributed to a synergistic effect.

3.4.1.3 Clinical Studies

Evidence regarding anxiolytic effects of *C. asiatica* is somewhat scarce, although research interest has increased in recent years. In a systematic review, Ernst [58] found one study of *C. asiatica* that met search criteria. It was therefore stated that only preliminary data are available for this herb. Similarly, in a review including case reports, open-label and placebo-controlled trials, Baek and colleagues [45] reported that there is a scarcity of scientific evidence for the use of *C. asiatica* in the treatment of anxiety and insomnia. However, positive effects of *C. asiatica* on anxiety and general well-being have been demonstrated in a select number of human trials, providing a basis for further research.

In a small, double-blind RCT investigating acute effects on the acoustic startle response (ASR), 40 healthy participants were randomised to receive either 12 g *C. asiatica* or placebo. After 30 and 60 min, ASR amplitude was found to be significantly decreased for *C. asiatica* compared to placebo, although changes to self-rated anxiety were non-significant [48]. Considering that such a large dose of *C. asiatica* was administered, it is questionable as to whether this would be safe or effective long-term. Studies of the chronic effects of *C. asiatica* have used much lower doses, such as the 750 mg daily dose used by Wattanathorn and colleagues [59] who reported improved mood and cognitive function in an elderly population. However, in an RCT by Carlson and colleagues [60] which utilised only 68 mg *C. asiatica* in conjunction with Gingko biloba and fish oil, no treatment effect was reported in relation to overall Quality of Life (SF-36) scores in healthy older participants. It should be noted, however, that high baseline scores on the SF-36 were reported for participants in this study, suggesting that improvements may be range-limited.

With regard to clinical studies of *C. asiatica*, one open-label study was found with 33 participants diagnosed with Generalised Anxiety Disorder (GAD). *C. asiatica* leaf extract 500 mg BID was administered for 8 weeks. At the end of the study period, anxiety was significantly reduced, and stress and depression ratings were also reduced, as measured using the SF-36, Hamilton's Brief Psychiatric Rating Scale (BPRS) and the State-Trait Anxiety Inventory (STAI) [61].

3.4.1.4 Safety

The recommended adult daily dose of total triterpenoid fraction of *Centella asiatica* extracts standardised for asiaticoside, Asiatic acid and madecassic acid is 60–120 mg, and for crude herb the recommended daily dose is 0.5–6 g [63]. *C. asiatica* has been shown to be safe when administered in combination with Gingko Biloba and Docosahexanoic Acid (DHA). Participants receiving this combination formula experienced no significant differences from placebo in platelet function or experience of adverse events, and adverse events reported were minor [60]. However, some mild side effects have been reported in other trials, including skin reactions and gastrointestinal upset [45]. In addition, three cases of jaundice with elevated liver enzymes were reported in Argentina following *C. asiatica* consumption for 20–60 days [62], although the dosage and standardisation of the consumed extract is unknown, and the patients recovered on discontinuation. As there is limited knowledge regarding long-term safety of *C. asiatica* consumption or the safety during breastfeeding, it is recommended that use of *C. asiatica* should not exceed 6 weeks and that nursing mothers should refrain from using this herb [50].

3.5 Siberian Ginseng (*Eleutherococcus senticosus*)

Siberian Ginseng (*Eleutherococcus senticosus*) belongs to the Araliaceae family, a family native to Asia, the Malay peninsula, Polynesia, Europe, North Africa and the Americas [64]. According to Chinese medical records, *E. senticosus* has been used for over two centuries to increase vitality and energy, and has also been used by Russian cosmonauts to aid with adaptation to life stressors in space [3]. Davydov and Krikorian [65] reported that *E. senticosus* was first introduced to Europe as an adaptogen and ergogen (referring to increased potential for work output) through encounters with Soviet trainers and athletes who had incorporated it into their training regimes.

3.5.1 Mechanism of Action

The adaptogenic effects of *E. senticosus* are thought to be due to the capacity of its secondary metabolites to exert protective and inhibitory actions against free radicals [65]. *E. senticosus* roots contain the active constituents eleutherosides, triterpenoid-saponins and glycans, while the leaves contain hyperoside, a flavanol glycoside which has been reported to be an effective sedative [66]. Eleutherosides have demonstrated ability to improve carbohydrate metabolism and energy provision and to increase synthesis of protein and nucleic acids [67]. It is thought that these factors may prevent the exhaustion stage of the stress response, although more evidence is needed [3]. In addition, *E. senticosus* may exert neuroprotective, hepatoprotective and cardioprotective activity [67]. In times of chronic stress, repeated *E. senticosus* administration has been found to engage the HPA axis, enabling the body to adapt to repeated stressors by balancing the switch-on and switch-off stress responses [67].

It has been postulated that the stimulating single-dose effect of *E. senticosus* may be due to the relatively high amounts of phenolic 28 compounds such as phenylpropane or phenylethane derivatives, as high amounts of these compounds are also found in other adaptogens with demonstrated single-dose effects such as *R. rosea* and *S. chinensis*.These compounds are structurally similar to the catecholamines, and are thought to play roles in the sympathoadrenal and central nervous systems [68]. In contrast, the adaptogenic effect of repeated administration is thought to be due to accumulated levels of tetracyclic triterpenes that are structurally similar to corticosteroids, and alter HPA-axis activity [68].

3.5.2 Preclinical Studies

E. senticosus has been shown to protect against physiological markers of stress. In a study by Mills and Bone [69], adrenal hypertrophy and adrenal ascorbic acid depletion (indicators of stress) were significantly reduced in rodents following *E. senticosus* treatment. These effects allow the organism to better withstand prolonged stress [3]. In addition, increased endurance during a forced swim test in mice has been demonstrated following administration of both hyperoside from *E.senticosus* leaf [66] and ADAPT-232, a combination of extracts *E. senticosus*, *R. rosea* and *S. chinensis* [70].

3.5.3 Clinical Studies

Many of the human clinical trials data regarding the adaptogenic effects of *E. senticosus* have been conducted in the Soviet Union and have not been published in English language journals. Farnsworth and colleagues [71] reviewed many of these studies which included participants from 19 to 72 years. It was concluded that *E. senticosus* increases the ability to adapt to adverse physical conditions, improves mental performance and enables higher quality of work. Davydov and Krikorian [65] also conducted a review of the Russian literature and reported that humans who were administered *E. senticosus* demonstrated superior performance on stressful tasks in comparison to those administered *Panax ginseng* and placebo.

Early research suggested that *E. senticosus* was inactive when administered as a daily dose of tea [72]. However, in a follow-up study Berdyshev [73] reported that *E. senticosus* improved mental performance in a correction test in a sample of 357 sailors on night duty. Moreover, several physiological effects were observed, such as increased intensity of metabolic processes and improved endurance to hypoxia (breathing of CO_2). A dose of 4 mL was found to be the most effective in improving work ability, whilst a higher dose of 8 mL did not show any further improvement and in fact resulted in a worsening of some objective and subjective measures, such as feeling sleepy [73].

More recently, Western studies have been conducted and published in English. In a double-blind RCT, 45 volunteers were administered *E. senticosus* or placebo for 30 days. Reduced heart rate in response to a Stroop Colour-Word stressor was found for *E. senticosus* (2 vials/day) compared with placebo. Females, but not males, receiving *E. senticosus* also showed reduced systolic blood pressure compared with placebo. These findings suggest that *E. senticosus* may be useful for reducing the stress response, perhaps more so in females [74]. In a 2-month RCT examining the effects of *E. senticosus* (four 500 mg capsules per day, standardised to 2.24 mg eleutherosides and equivalent to a dried root dosage of 2–4 g per day) in 96 participants suffering from chronic fatigue, similar reductions in fatigue were observed for both *E. senticosus* and placebo, suggesting no beneficial effect of the herbal preparation. However, sub-group analysis revealed that treatment with *E. senticosus* was effective for subjects with less severe fatigue at 2 months, a finding that is worthy of further investigation [75].

However, in a recent study investigating the effectiveness of *E. senticosus* compared with 2-day professional stress management training, 120 mg/day *E. senticosus* for 8 weeks was not found to be significantly superior on any parameter, including cognitive performance, subjective ratings of feeling stressed, mood and quality of life, and cortisol awakening response in participants suffering from low energy and reduced working capacity [76]. Combining *E. senticosus* with stress management training resulted in significantly improved outcomes compared with *E. senticosus* alone, but not compared with stress management training alone. These findings indicate that adding *E. senticosus* treatment to stress management training may not be beneficial, and that stress management training alone may be just as effective.

Considering these findings, it is interesting to note that *E. senticosus* has been theorised to act in different ways to support the body depending on stressor severity. It has been suggested that when stress levels are below a certain threshold and allostatic load is such that responses have become inadequate, the stress response is increased by *E. senticosus*. Conversely, when chronic stress levels are above a certain threshold the stress response is reduced through the triggering of negative feedback systems [67]. Therefore, according to this theory the stress-reducing effects of *E. senticosus* may only become apparent when chronic stress levels are high. During times of chronic stress it appears that maximal effects of *E. senticosus* are achieved around 4 weeks but do not persist beyond 8 weeks. Therefore, treatment has been typically given for 6–8 weeks, with a break of 1–2 weeks before recommencing [67]. It is noted that the studies included in this review examine only chronic effects of *E. senticosus*; therefore, further studies are required to assess the effects of acute administration.

3.6 Schisandra (*Schisandra chinensis*)

Schisandra (*Schisandra chinensis*) is a deciduous vine that grows in northern China, Japan, Korea and far-eastern Russia. The berries have been widely used in Traditional Chinese Medicine alongside other herbs to increase resistance to physical and emotional stressors, in addition to being used for ailments such as mouth dryness, coughs, dysentery and insomnia in China, Korea and Japan [77]. The tonic and stimulatory effects of *S. chinensis* were reported in several Soviet Union WWII military journals, and the berries and seeds were used by Nanai hunters for reasons such as reducing hunger, thirst and exhaustion (see [78], for a review).

3.6.1 Mechanism of Action

The chemical composition of *S. chinensis* fruit is still not fully known [79]; however, the key biologically active constituents are believed to be dibenzocyclooctenelignans, such as schisandrin and gomisin [80]. *S. chinensis* fruits are also rich in polysaccharides, monosaccharides, vitamins, phytosterols, organic acids and bioelements. Schisandrin has been shown to produce beneficial sedative effects, possibly through modification of the serotonergic system [81], whilst polysaccharides may also raise neurotransmitter levels [82, 83].

3.6.2 Preclinical Studies

Animal studies have demonstrated a number of beneficial treatment effects associated with *S. chinensis* including increased physical working capacity (e.g. [84–86], anti-stress effects (Barnaulov and Shanin [87]; in [88]), anxiolytic effects [89] and protection against toxicity [88, 90, 91]. Xia et al. [92] reported that *S. chinensis* decreased stress-induced elevation of corticotropin-releasing hormone and peripheral corticosterone levels, effects that they suggest may demonstrate an anti-stress effect of *S. chinensis* via balancing of the HPA axis. Wu et al. [93] similarly reported an attenuation of the stress-induced increase in corticosterone levels, as well as increased time spent in the arms of an EPM, following 3 days treatment with aqueous *S. chinensis* extract.

3.6.3 Clinical Studies

Similar to *E. senticosus*, the majority of clinical studies of *S. chinensis* have been conducted in Russia and the publications have often not been translated into English. Panossian and colleagues [4, 43, 78, 88], however, have conducted some comprehensive reviews of this literature and concluded that *S. chinensis* has stimulating properties and acts as an adaptogen following single-dose administration. Some of the studies included in these reviews are discussed below.

In a series of early studies, Lebedev and others [94–97] investigated the effects of *S. chinensis* on mental working capacity in fatigued individuals. Improvements were seen following treatment in terms of the number of errors made and amount of work performed. Gubchenko and Fruentov [98] also reported superior attention and memory functions following an acute dose of *S. chinensis* compared with placebo. The same authors conducted a chronic study in pilots, who were tested both pre- and post-flight on a number of outcomes including attention and memory functions, sensorimotor response and precision. Ten days' treatment with *S. chinensis* tincture resulted in significant improvements in these parameters compared with placebo [99].

Grigorenko and Berdyshev [72] examined the effects of a single daily dose of *S. chinensis* tea in sailors on night shift. For the first 7–10 days, the treatment had a tonic effect on those keeping watch; however, continuous use of the tea over 2–3 weeks led to some participants experiencing sleeplessness and excitability. In a further study, Berdyshev [73] conducted a placebo-controlled crossover trial to investigate single-dose administration of both *S. chinensis* and *E. senticosus* in 357 sailors on watch duty. *S. chinensis* was reported to improve working ability parameters as well as having several physiological effects such as increased cardiovascular and respiratory activity, increased activity of the CNS at night and intensified oxidation-reduction and metabolic processes [73]. Based on these findings the author concluded that *S. chinensis* acts as a mild stimulant.

The adaptogenic effects of *S. chinensis* have been studied in athletes together with the effects of *Bryonia alba*. In a placebo-controlled RCT, Panossian and colleagues [100] measured the content of nitric oxide (NO) and cortisol in blood and saliva before and after herbal treatment, as well as before and after exercise. Both herbs significantly increased basal levels of salivary NO compared with placebo and reduced the effect of heavy physical exercise on increasing NO. These findings were accompanied by an increase of physical performance, which the authors postulated may be due to their stimulatory effect on NO production, which adapts the organism to heavy physical exercise [100].

3.6.4 Safety

Findings from early studies suggest minimal side effects of *S. chinensis* in healthy humans. In doses of 3.6 mg up to 20 mg only four out of 153 subjects experienced excitation and three reported experiencing depression [96]. In a large-scale study of 1,200 patients, Masyuk (1949; in [88]) reported that 8 months' treatment with infusions of Schizandra leaves resulted in no dependency and no significant adverse events. Only 3.3 % of patients ceased taking the treatment due to excitation. More recently, Kormosh and colleagues [101] reported no herb–drug interactions in cancer patients taking *S. chinensis*.

3.7 Combination Preparations

In addition to the evidence suggesting beneficial effects of individual adaptogens, efficacy of standardised combinations of adaptogens has been demonstrated in numerous studies. ADAPT-232 is a combination of extracts of roots of *R. rosea*, berries of *S. chinensis* and roots of *E. senticosus* (3 mg *R. rosea*, 4 mg *S. chinensis*, 3 mg *E. senticosus*). ADAPT-232 tablets are standardised with respect to rhodioloside (0.32 %), rosavin (0.5 %), tyrosol (0.05 %), schizandrin (0.37 %), γ-schizandrin (0.24 %) and eleutherosides B and E (0.15 %). The Centre for Space Medicine of the Institute of Medicinal and Biological Problems and the Moscow Aviation Institute have conducted a series of studies examining the adaptogenic effects of ADAPT-232. In these studies, ADAPT-232 has been shown to improve performance in terms of both speed and precision in conditions simulating those encountered on space stations. These effects were most pronounced against a background of high fatigue, and were most marked in complicated tests and under extreme conditions. Compared with placebo, fewer mistakes were made 4 h after administration and working capacity was increased 1.5 and 4 h after administration [102, 103].

In a sample of women experiencing long-term stress, a single 270 mg dose of ADAPT-232 resulted in significantly improved attention, speed and accuracy 2 h post-dose compared with placebo [104]. ADAPT-232 has also been shown to improve quality of life and increase mental performance in patients recovering from pneumonia, whilst decreasing the acute phase of the illness by 2 days [105]. According to Panossian and Wikman [78] ADAPT-232 works as a "stress vaccine"; reducing levels of nitric oxide, cortisol and c-Jun N-terminal protein kinase (JNK) under stress, as well as stimulating expression of the heat shock protein Hsp70, which enhances the repair of damaged proteins and increases levels of adenosine triphosphate (ATP) back to normal levels. Rodelim is a different combination of extracts of the same plants and has also shown improvements in mental working capacity in healthy volunteers. Roslyakova and colleagues [106] found that an acute dose of 100 mg Rodelim administered to fatigued participants resulted in improved mental working capacity in computer and correction tests.

3.7.1 Clinical Considerations

The adaptogens discussed in this chapter all have at least some demonstrated evidence for the reduction of stress and anxiety. With the exception of *S. chinensis*, all these herbs appear to have beneficial effects when administered chronically or in repeated low doses. The evidence for chronic use of WS is particularly strong, although there may be more evidence for other adaptogens that is not currently available for review in English. In the case of *S. chinensis*, repeated administration up to 10 days may be effective, but longer-term use may result in detrimental effects, such as sleeplessness. Chronic use of this herb is therefore not recommended, particularly for patients experiencing anxiety with insomnia. Evidence regarding the acute effects of WS and *E. senticosus* is somewhat lacking; however, it appears that the other adaptogens discussed in this chapter may have beneficial effects following single-dose administration. In particular, *R. rosea* appears to be a promising treatment in the event that acute anxiolytic effects are required.

The majority of research that has been undertaken on these compounds has involved healthy non-clinical populations. However, some adaptogens have demonstrated efficacy in clinical populations. In particular, WS has been shown to significantly reduce symptoms in patients experiencing clinically significant anxiety symptoms, as well as patients with OCD. Preliminary data exist for the use of *R. rosea* and *C. asiatica* in the treatment of GAD, although larger, placebo-controlled RCTs are required to further corroborate these initial findings. In addition, further trials will be needed to determine whether adaptogens may be a viable treatment for anxiety disorders other than GAD, such as social anxiety disorder and panic disorder.

When prescribing any medication, including natural therapies, it is important to consider the evidence regarding safety. The majority of evidence suggests only minor side effects associated with the use of adaptogens in most individuals. However, adaptogens have been reported to have unwanted excitatory effects for some people; therefore, caution should be used when administering these compounds to patients suffering with insomnia or bipolar disorder. In addition, *C. asiatica* may have effects on liver function, and chronic consumption was found to result in jaundice in one study. Whilst further research is needed to determine whether these side effects are indeed due to *C. asiatica* consumption, it is recommended that liver function is monitored if this herb is used chronically.

Whilst adaptogens appear to be safe in the majority of cases, data are also limited regarding interactions with pharmaceutical drugs. *R. rosea* may inhibit proteins affecting drug metabolism, thereby increasing the bioavailability of some drugs. Caution should therefore be applied when prescribing this herb. However, there is currently no evidence to suggest that *R. rosea* is unsafe when used alongside other treatments. With regard to WS, one study found it to be safe and well-tolerated when administered as an adjunct to SSRIs. Further research is needed to determine whether adaptogens may be beneficial when prescribed alongside psychotherapies, such as CBT, or whether they would provide no further benefit as found in a study by Schaffler and colleagues [75].

In summary, further research is required in order to more clearly determine the optimal dose and durations of treatment for each of the adaptogens discussed. However, preliminary data suggest that this class of natural medicines may have efficacy in the reduction of stress and anxiety, particulary in the context of increased task demands. WS and *R. rosea* appear to be particularly effective for chronic and acute administration, respectively, and may also have potential application in the treatment of clinically significant anxiety.

References

1. Farrell AK, Simpson JA. Effects of relationship functioning on the biological experience of stress and physical health. Curr Opin Psychiatry. 2017;13:49–53.
2. Burton L, Westen D, Kowalski R. Psychology. 3rd Australian and New Zealand ed. Milton: Wiley Australia; 2012.
3. Provino R. The role of adaptogens in stress management. Australian J Med Herbalism. 2010;22(2):41–9.
4. Panossian A, Wikman G. Evidence-based efficacy of adaptogens in fatigue, and molecular mechanisms related to their stress-protective activity. Curr Clin Pharmacol. 2009;4(3):198–219.
5. Darbinyan V et al. *Rhodiolarosea* in stress induced fatigue – a double blind cross-over study of a standardized extract SHR-5 with a repeated low-dose regimen on the mental performance of healthy physicians during night duty. Phytomedicine. 2000;7(5):365–71.
6. Kulkarni SK, Dhir A. *Withaniasomnifera*: an Indian ginseng. Prog Neuropsychopharmacol Biol Psychiatry. 2008;32(5):1093–105.
7. Alramadhan E et al. Dietary and botanical anxiolytics. Med Sci Monit. 2012;18(4):RA40–8.

8. Mishra LC, Singh BB, Dagenais S. Scientific basis for the therapeutic use of *Withaniasomnifera* (ashwagandha): a review. Altern Med Rev. 2000;5(4):334–46.
9. Schliebs R et al. Systemic administration of defined extracts from *Withaniasomnifera* (Indian Ginseng) and Shilajit differentially affects cholinergic but not glutamatergic and gabaergic markers in rat brain. Neurochem Int. 1997;30(2):181–90.
10. Matsuda H et al. Structures of withanosides I, II, III, IV, V, VI, and VII, new withanolide glycosides, from the roots of Indian *Withaniasomnifera* DUNAL. and inhibitory activity for tachyphylaxis to clonidine in isolated guinea-pig ileum. Bioorg Med Chem. 2001;9(6):1499–507.
11. Kulkarni S et al. GABA receptor mediated anticonvulsant action of *Withaniasomnifera* root extract. Indian Drugs. 1993;30(7):305–12.
12. Mehta A et al. Pharmacological effects of *Withaniasomnifera* root extract on GABAA receptor complex. Indian J Med Res. 1991;94:312–5.
13. Bhattacharya SK, Muruganandam AV. Adaptogenic activity of *Withaniasomnifera*: an experimental study using a rat model of chronic stress. Pharmacol Biochem Behav. 2003;75(3):547–55.
14. Bhattacharya SK et al. Anti-stress activity of sitoindosides VII and VIII, new acylsterylglucosides from *Withaniasomnifera*. Phytother Res. 1987;1(1):32–7.
15. Archana R, Namasivayam A. Antistressor effect of *Withaniasomnifera*. J Ethnopharmacol. 1998;64(1):91–3.
16. Dadkar VN, Ranadive N, Dhar H. Evaluation of antistress (adaptogen) activity of *Withaniasomnifera* (ashwagandha).Ind J Clin Bio Chem. 1987;2:101–8.
17. Grandhi A, Mujumdar AM, Patwardhan B. A comparative pharmacological investigation of Ashwagandha and Ginseng. J Ethnopharmacol. 1994;44(3):131–5.
18. Bhattacharya SK et al. Anxiolytic-antidepressant activity of *Withaniasomnifera* glycowithanolides: an experimental study. Phytomedicine. 2000;7(6):463–9.
19. Pratte MA et al. An alternative treatment for anxiety: a systematic review of human trial results reported for the Ayurvedic Herb Ashwagandha (*Withaniasomnifera*). J Altern Complement Med. 2014;20(12):901–8.
20. Andrade C et al. A double-blind, placebo-controlled evaluation of the anxiolytic efficacy ff an ethanolic extract of *Withaniasomnifera*. Indian JPsychiatry. 2000;42(3):295.
21. Auddy B, Hazra PJ, Mitra PA. A standardized *Withaniasomnifera* extract significantly reduces stress-related parameters in chronically stressed humans: a double-blind, randomized, placebo-controlled study. J Am Nutraceutical Assoc. 2008;11:50–6.
22. Cooley K et al. Naturopathic care for anxiety: a randomized controlled trial ISRCTN78958974. PLoS One. 2009;4(8):e6628.
23. Chandrasekhar K, Kapoor J, Anishetty S. A prospective, randomized double-blind, placebo-controlled study of safety and efficacy of a high-concentration full-spectrum extract of Ashwagandha root in reducing stress and anxiety in adults. Indian J Psychol Med. 2012;34(3):255–62.
24. SudKhyati S, Anup BT. A randomized double blind placebo controlled study of ashwagandha on generalized anxiety disorder. IntAyurvedic Med J. 2013;1:1–7.
25. Jahanbakhsh SP et al. Evaluation of the efficacy of *Withaniasomnifera* (Ashwagandha) root extract in patients with obsessive-compulsive disorder: a randomized double-blind placebo-controlled trial. Complement Ther Med. 2016;27:25–9.
26. Kushwaha S, Betsy A, Chawla P. Effect of Ashwagandha (*Withaniasomnifera*) root powder supplementation in treatment of hypertension. Stud Ethno-Med. 2012;6(2):111–5.
27. TalbottSM,KraemerWJ.The cortisol connection: why stress makes you fat and ruins your health-and what you can do about it. Alameda, CA: Hunter House; 2007.
28. Mell C. Dyes, tannins, perfumes, and medicines from *Rhodiolarosea*. Textile Colorist. 1938;60(715):483–4.
29. Panossian A, Wikman G, Sarris J. Rosenroot (*Rhodiolarosea*): traditional use, chemical composition, pharmacology and clinical efficacy. Phytomedicine. 2010;17(7):481–93.

30. Shevtsov VA et al. A randomized trial of two different doses of a SHR-5 *Rhodiolarosea* extract versus placebo and control of capacity for mental work. Phytomedicine. 2003;10(2-3):95–105.
31. Ming DS et al. Bioactive compounds from *Rhodiolarosea* (Crassulaceae). Phytother Res. 2005;19(9):740–3.
32. Aksyonova R. The stimulating and adaptogenic effect of a purified *Rhodiolarosea* preparation–rhodosine. In: Stimulants of the central nervous system. Tomsk; 1966. p. 77–9.
33. Saratikov A. Golden root (*Rhodiolarosea*). Tomsk: Russia; 1974.
34. Sokolov SY et al. Studies of neurotropic activity of new agents isolated from Rodiola-rosea. Khimiko-Farmatsevticheskii Zhurnal. 1985;19(11):1367–71.
35. Petkov VD et al. Effects of alcohol aqueous extract from *Rhodiolarosea* L. roots on learning and memory. Acta Physiol Pharmacol Bulg. 1986;12(1):3–16.
36. Norr H. Phytochemical and pharmacological Investigations of the Adaptogens: *Eleutherococcussenticosus*, *Ocimum sanctum*, *Codonopsispilosula*, *Rhodiolarosea* and Rhodiola crenulata. Û Ludwig Maximilians University. Û Muenchen; 1993. p. 228.
37. Wagner H, Nörr H, Winterhoff H. Plant adaptogens. Phytomedicine. 1994;1(1):63–76.
38. Olsson EM, von Schéele B, Panossian AG. A randomised, double-blind, placebo-controlled, parallel-group study of the standardised extract shr-5 of the roots of *Rhodiolarosea* in the treatment of subjects with stress-related fatigue. Planta Med. 2009;75(2):105.
39. Van Diermen D et al. Monoamine oxidase inhibition by *Rhodiolarosea* L. roots. J Ethnopharmacol. 2009;122(2):397–401.
40. Stancheva S, Mosharrof A. Effect of the extract of Rhodiola-rosea L on the content of the brain biogenic monoamines. Dokladi Na Bolgarskata Akademiya Na Naukite. 1987;40(6):85–7.
41. Kelly GS. *Rhodiolarosea*: a possible plant adaptogen. Altern Med Rev. 2001;6(3):293–302.
42. Azizov AP, Seifulla RD. The effect of elton, leveton, phytoton, and adapton on the working capacity of experimental animals. Geogr Rev. 1998;88(3):63.
43. Panossian A, Wagner H. Stimulating effect of adaptogens: an overview with particular reference to their efficacy following single dose administration. Phytother Res. 2005;19(10):819–38.
44. Bystritsky A, Kerwin L, Feusner JD. A pilot study of *Rhodiolarosea* (Rhodax®) for generalized anxiety disorder (GAD). J Altern Complement Med. 2008;14(2):175–80.
45. Baek JH, Nierenberg AA, Kinrys G. Clinical applications of herbal medicines for anxiety and insomnia; targeting patients with bipolar disorder. Aust N Z J Psychiatry. 2014;48(8):705–15.
46. Hellum BH et al. Potent in vitro inhibition of CYP3A4 and P-glycoprotein by *Rhodiolarosea*. Planta Med. 2010;76(4):331–8.
47. Head KA, Kelly GS. Nutrients and botanicals for treatment of stress: adrenal fatigue, neurotransmitter imbalance, anxiety, and restless sleep. Altern Med Rev. 2009;14(2):114–40.
48. Bradwejn J et al. A double-blind, placebo-controlled study on the effects of Gotu Kola (*Centellaasiatica*) on acoustic startle response in healthy subjects. J Clin Psychopharmacol. 2000;20(6):680–4.
49. Wijeweera P et al. Evaluation of anxiolytic properties of Gotukola – (*Centellaasiatica*) extracts and asiaticoside in rat behavioral models. Phytomedicine. 2006;13(9–10):668–76.
50. Gohil KJ, Patel JA, Gajjar AK. Pharmacological review on *Centellaasiatica*: a potential herbal cure-all. Indian J Pharm Sci. 2010;72(5):546–56.
51. Grimaldi R et al. Pharmacokinetics of the total triterpenic fraction of *Centellaasiatica* after single and multiple administrations to healthy volunteers. A new assay for asiatic acid. J Ethnopharmacol. 1990;28(2):235–41.
52. Chen Y et al. Effects of total triterpenes of *Centellaasiatica* on the corticosterone levels in serum and contents of monoamine in depression rat brain. Zhong Yao Cai (Zhongyaocai, Journal of Chinese Medicinal Materials). 2005;28(6):492–6.
53. Chatterjee TK et al. Effects of plant extract *Centellaasiatica* (Linn.) on cold restraint stress ulcer in rats. Indian J Exp Biol. 1992;30(10):889–91.

54. Awad R et al. Effects of traditionally used anxiolytic botanicals on enzymes of the γ-aminobutyric acid (GABA) system. Can J Physiol Pharmacol. 2007;85(9):933–42.
55. Ceremuga TE et al. Evaluation of the anxiolytic and antidepressant effects of asiatic acid, a compound from Gotu kola or *Centellaasiatica*, in the male Sprague Dawley rat. AANA J. 2015;83(2):91–8.
56. Ramaswamy A, Periyasamy S, Basu N. Pharmacological studies on Centella asaitica Linn. (Brahma manduki)(no Umbelliferae). J Res Indian Med. 1970;4:160–75.
57. Chen SW et al. Anxiolytic-like effect of asiaticoside in mice. Pharmacol Biochem Behav. 2006;85(2):339–44.
58. Ernst E. Herbal remedies for anxiety – a systematic review of controlled clinical trials. Phytomedicine. 2006;13(3):205–8.
59. Wattanathorn J et al. Positive modulation of cognition and mood in the healthy elderly volunteer following the administration of *Centellaasiatica*. J Ethnopharmacol. 2008;116(2):325–32.
60. Carlson JJ et al. Safety and efficacy of a ginkgo biloba-containing dietary supplement on cognitive function, quality of life, and platelet function in healthy, cognitively intact older adults. J Am Diet Assoc. 2007;107(3):422–32.
61. Jana U et al. A clinical study on the management of generalized anxiety disorder with *Centellaasiatica*. Nepal Med CollJournal (NMCJ). 2010;12(1):8–11.
62. Jorge OA, Jorge AD. Hepatotoxicity associated with the ingestion of *Centellaasiatica*. Rev Esp Enferm Dig. 2005;97(2):115–24.
63. Turton S. *Centellaasiatica*. Australian J Herbal Med. 1993;5(3):57–61.
64. Wielgorskaya T, Takhtadzhi͡an AL. Dictionary of generic names of seed plants. New York: Columbia University Press; 1995.
65. Davydov M, Krikorian AD. *Eleutherococcussenticosus* (Rupr. and Maxim.) Maxim. (Araliaceae) as an adaptogen: a closer look. J Ethnopharmacol. 2000;72(3):345–93.
66. Takeshi D, Sansei N, Yoshihisa N. Constituents and pharmacological effects of Eucommia and Siberian ginseng. Acta Pharmacol Sin. 2001;22:1057–70.
67. Oates L. Siberian ginseng *Eleutherococcussenticosus*. J Complement Med. 2008;7(4):44–7 , +67.
68. Pawar VS, Shivakumar H. A current status of adaptogens: natural remedy to stress. Asian Pac J Trop Dis. 2012;2(Suppl1):S480–90.
69. Mills S, Bone K. Principles and practice of phytotherapy. London: Churchill livigstone; 2000.
70. Panossian A et al. Adaptogens exert a stress-protective effect by modulation of expression of molecular chaperones. Phytomedicine. 2009;16(6):617–22.
71. FarnsworthNet al. Siberian ginseng (*Eleutherococcussenticosus*): current status as an adaptogen.In: Wagner H, Hikino H, Farnsworth NR, editors. Economic and medicinal plant research, 1985.
72. Grigorenko G,Berdishev V. The use of tonic drinks and drugs increasing working capacity of sailors during night shifts. In Abstract Book of the Scientific Practical Conference on Medical and Social Aspects of the "Man-Ocean" Problem ,Vladivostok, Russia; 1988.
73. Berdyshev V. Some specific effects of single doses of adaptogens. Valeology: diagnosis, means and practice in health care. IntCollection SciPapers. 1995;2:105–17.
74. Facchinetti F, Neri I, Tarabusi M. *Eleutherococcussenticosus* reduces cardiovascular stress response in healthy subjects: a randomized, placebo-controlled trial. Stress Health. 2002;18(1):11–7.
75. Hartz A et al. Randomized controlled trial of Siberian ginseng for chronic fatigue. Psychol Med. 2004;34(01):51–61.
76. Schaffler K, Wolf OT, Burkart M. No benefit adding *Eleutherococcussenticosus* to stress management training in stress-related fatigue/weakness, impaired work or concentration, a randomized controlled study. Pharmacopsychiatry. 2013;46(5):181–90.
77. Hung TM et al. Acetylcholinesterase inhibitory effect of lignans isolated fromSchizandra chinensis. Arch Pharm Res. 2007;30(6):685–90.

78. Panossian A, Wikman G. Effects of adaptogens on the central nervous system and the molecular mechanisms associated with their stress—protective activity. Pharmaceuticals. 2010;3(1):188–224.
79. Szopa A, Ekiert R, Ekiert H. Current knowledge of Schisandra Chinensis. Phytochemsitry reviews. 2016:1–24.
80. Bone K. A clinical guide to blending liquid herbs: herbal formulations for the individual patient. London: Elsevier Health Sciences; 2003.
81. Zhang C et al. Pharmacological evaluation of sedative and hypnotic effects of schizandrin through the modification of pentobarbital-induced sleep behaviors in mice. Eur J Pharmacol. 2014;744:157–63.
82. Chen Y et al. An immunostimulatory polysaccharide (SCP-IIa) from the fruit of Schisandra chinensis (Turcz.) Baill. Int J Biol Macromol. 2012;50(3):844–8.
83. Zhao T et al. Antitumor and immunomodulatory activity of a water-soluble low molecular weight polysaccharide from Schisandra chinensis (Turcz.) Baill. Food Chem Toxicol. 2013;55:609–16.
84. Lupandin A et al. On the adaptogenic effect of Schizandra and other adaptogens.In Brekhman II, Fruentov NK, editors. Syktyvkar: acute and chronic stress. VL Komarov's Far East Branch of USSR Academy of Science; 1986. p. 86–90.
85. Lupandin A, Ovsyanikova V. Increasing resistance to unfavourable factors under the effect of Schizandrachinensis extract. In: Brekhman II editor. Physiological mechanisms of adaptation. Russia: Ivanovo State University; 1986. p. 92–7.
86. Lupandin A. The role of catecholaminergic synapses in the mechanisms of the formation of adaptation with the participation of polyphenol adaptogens. Fiziologicheskii zhurnal SSSR imeni IM Sechenova. 1989;75(8):1082–8.
87. Barnaulov OD, Shanin SN. Stress-limiting effect of phytopreparations: endocrine system and detrimental environmental factors. In: Abstracts of the Fourth All-Union Conference, November 1991. Ministry of Health of USSR, Moscow, p. 27.
88. Panossian A, Wikman G. Pharmacology of Schisandra chinensis Bail.: an overview of Russian research and uses in medicine. J Ethnopharmacol. 2008;118(2):183–212.
89. Chen W-W et al. Pharmacological studies on the anxiolytic effect of standardized Schisandra lignans extract on restraint-stressed mice. Phytomedicine. 2011;18(13):1144–7.
90. Kim SR et al. Dibenzocyclooctadiene lignans from Schisandra chinensis protect primary cultures of rat cortical cells from glutamate-induced toxicity. J Neurosci Res. 2004;76(3):397–405.
91. You JS, Pan TL, Hou YC. Schisandra chinensis protects against adriamycin-induced cardiotoxicity in rats. Chang Gung Med J. 2006;29(1):63–70.
92. Xia N et al. Schisandra chinensis and *Rhodiolarosea* exert an anti-stress effect on the HPA axis and reduce hypothalamic c-Fos expression in rats subjected to repeated stress. Exp Ther Med. 2016;11(1):353–9.
93. Wu YY et al. Effects of the aqueous extract of Schizandra chinensis fruit on ethanol withdrawal-induced anxiety in rats. Chin Med J (Engl). 2014;127(10):1935–40.
94. Lebedev A. Comparative evaluation of the stimulating effect of various Schizandra products. In Materials for the study of stimulants and tonics from Ginseng and Schizandra roots. Issue 1. Vladivostok: Komarovs' Far East Branch of USSR Academy of Science. 1951. p. 103–8.
95. Lebedev A. Some materials on the pharmacology of schizandrin. Issue 1. Vladivostok: Komarovs' Far East Branch of USSR Academy of Science. 1951. p. 109–17.
96. Lebedev A. Schizandrin—a new stimulant from Schizandrachinensis fruits. Summary of Thesis for a Candidate's Degree in Medicine, Tashkent; 1967.
97. Kochmareva L. The effect of Schizandrachinensis and Ginseng on processes of concentration. In: Lazarev (ed.). Materials for the study of Ginseng and Leningrad: V. L. Komarov's Far East Branch of USSR Academy of Science. 1958. p. 12–17.

98. Gubchenko P, Fruentov N. A comparative study of stimulating effect of adaptogenic agents prepared from some far-eastern plants. New data on Eleutherococcus and other adaptogens. Vladivostok: USSR Academy of Science, Far East Science Center, Institute of Marin Biology; 1981. p. 18–25.
99. Gubchenko P, Fruentov N. Comparative study of the effectiveness of Eleutherococcus and other plant adaptogens as remedies for increasing the work capacity of flight personnel. In Newdata on Eleutherococcus: proceedings of the 2nd international symposium on Eleutherococcus (Moscow, 1984). Vladivostok: Far East Academy of Science of the USSR; 1986.
100. Panossian AG et al. Effects of heavy physical exercise and adaptogens on nitric oxide content in human saliva. Phytomedicine. 1999;6(1):17–26.
101. Kormosh N, Laktionov K, Antoshechkina M. Effect of a combination of extract from several plants on cell-mediated and humoral immunity of patients with advanced ovarian cancer. Phytother Res. 2006;20(5):424–5.
102. Bogatova RI et al. Evaluation of the effect of a single dose of phytoadaptogen on human's working ability during long-term isolation. Aviakosmicheskaia i ekologicheskaia meditsina(Aerospace and Environmental Medicine). 1997;31(4):51–4.
103. Bogatova R, Malozemov V. Experimental research on estimation of influence of single dose of phytoadaptogens on short memory. The report on Moscow: Institute of Medical and Biological Problems (IMBP). 1994. p. 1–151.
104. Aslanyan G et al. Double-blind, placebo-controlled, randomised study of single dose effects of ADAPT-232 on cognitive functions. Phytomedicine. 2010;17(7):494–9.
105. Narimanian M et al. Impact of Chisan® (ADAPT-232) on the quality-of-life and its efficacy as an adjuvant in the treatment of acute non-specific pneumonia. Phytomedicine. 2005;12(10):723–9.
106. Roslyakova N et al. The effect of single dose of Rodelim phytoadaptogen on the performance of operators under intensive activity. In Abstract book of scientific conference biologically active food supplements and natural medicines in prophylaxis, treatment and rehabilitation, Moscow, Russia; 2000.

Cognitive Anxiolytics

4

Genevieve Z. Steiner and Danielle C. Mathersul

4.1 Introduction

Cognitive deficits, such as poor concentration, attention, and memory, are common features of anxiety disorders, including generalised anxiety disorder (GAD), panic disorder (PD), and social anxiety disorder (SAD) [1–4]. First-line pharmacological treatments for anxiety disorders, particularly benzodiazepines, may compound these cognitive deficits due to their sedative actions [5, 6]. Complementary and alternative treatments with combined anxiolytic and cognitive-enhancing properties, hereto referred to as cognitive anxiolytics, would be beneficial to the field. The research outlined in this chapter details evidence on a range of herbs including *Bacopa monnieri*, *Ginkgo biloba*, *Melissa officinalis*, *Camellia sinensis*, *Salvia* spp., and *Rosmarinus officinalis* that have both cognitive-enhancing and anxiolytic properties. A range of mechanisms of action have been proposed to account for these effects including antioxidant, acetylcholinesterase (AChE) inhibition, increased cerebral blood flow (CBF), cholinergic enhancement (binding to both nicotinic and muscarinic receptors), and γ-aminobutyric acid (GABA) potentiation.

G.Z. Steiner (✉)
National Institute of Complementary Medicine, Western Sydney University, Locked Bag 1797, Penrith, NSW 2751, Australia
e-mail: G.Steiner@westernsydney.edu.au

D.C. Mathersul
War Related Illness and Injury Study Center, Veterans Affairs Palo Alto Health Care System, Palo Alto, CA 94304, USA

School of Medicine, Stanford University, Stanford, CA 94305, USA

Department of Psychology, University of Pennsylvania, Philadelphia, PA 19104, USA

D. Camfield et al. (eds.), *Evidence-Based Herbal and Nutritional Treatments for Anxiety in Psychiatric Disorders*, DOI 10.1007/978-3-319-42307-4_4

4.2 Brahmi (*Bacopa monnieri*)

4.2.1 Overview

Bacopa monnieri, known as Brahmi in Ayurvedic medicine, is a herb native to the northeast and southern regions of India, and is widely known for its memory-enhancing effects. Animal models and human trials have consistently demonstrated the nootropic properties of Brahmi. Recommendations as early as the sixth century AD suggest amelioration of a range of conditions, including lack of concentration and anxiety [7]; however, less research has examined Brahmi for both cognitive and anxiolytic effects. Traditionally, the leaves of the plant have been eaten fresh, fried in ghee, or juiced.

4.2.2 Mechanisms of Action

Brahmi is thought to have multiple possible actions including antioxidant, anxiolytic, anti-inflammatory, analgesic, metal chelating, and cholinergic effects [7], with the major active components being steroidal saponins, bacosides A and B. Evidence suggests that a range of mechanisms are involved including neuroprotection through redox and enzyme induction, choline acetyltransferase activation and/or AChE inhibition, increased CBF, and β-amyloid reduction [8]. Brahmi has also been shown to reduce norepinephrine in the hippocampus, hypothalamus, and cerebral cortex, which may indirectly modify acetylcholine (ACh) concentrations [9]. Anxiolytic effects are likely to result from strong antioxidant and anti-inflammatory actions after chronic administration.

There is less evidence on acute effects of Brahmi, leading some to conclude that actions are largely effective after chronic administration [10, 11]. In particular, the cognitive-enhancing effects of Brahmi are thought to result from cholinergic modulation (e.g., AChE inhibition), which is maximally effective after chronic administration [12]. This is similar for Brahmi's antioxidant properties, which have also been observed after chronic administration [13].

4.2.3 Evidence of Efficacy

4.2.3.1 Preclinical

Most animal work has focused on the cognitive-enhancing effects of Brahmi, particularly in disease models, with less work on its anxiolytic properties. For example, acute administration of Brahmi resulted in reduced cognitive deficits in the sub-chronic phencyclidine rat model of schizophrenia [14]. This was thought to result from a decrease in prefrontal cortex, striatum, and hippocampus NMDAR1 receptor density. Standardised Brahmi extract also improved spatial learning and memory retention, and increased hippocampal CA3 neuronal dendritic arborisation in rats [15]. One study showed a dose-related acute anxiolytic effect of standardised

Brahmi extract, comparable to lorazepam, without significantly reducing motor activity in CF strain male rats [16].

4.2.3.2 Acute Clinical Studies

There is some evidence from randomised controlled trials that Brahmi has both anxiolytic and cognitive-enhancing effects in humans. Most clinical studies have utilised standardised extracts, including CDRI 08, bacosides enriched standardised extract (BESEB), and Bacomind®. Acute 320 and 640 mg doses of standardised Brahmi extract (CDRI 08) led to improved cognition (Letter Search and Stroop tasks) and positive mood (contentedness and alertness, measured on a Visual Analogue Scale [VAS]), and reduced salivary cortisol in a double-blind, placebo-controlled cross-over study (n = 17) [17]. Further, acute administration of 320 or 640 mg of standardised Brahmi extract (CDRI 08) resulted in improved task performance on the Cognitive Demand Battery, but did not affect cardiovascular activity or task-induced ratings of stress and fatigue in a randomised, double-blind, placebo-controlled trial (n = 24) [11].

4.2.3.3 Chronic Clinical Studies

A 12-week randomised, double-blind, placebo-controlled trial (n = 54, M_{age} = 73.5 years) of 300 mg/day of standardised Brahmi extract (minimum 50 % bacosides A and B) or placebo found that Brahmi enhanced delayed word recall memory scores and Stroop task results, and decreased trait anxiety (State-Trait Anxiety Inventory [STAI]) *cf.* placebo in older men [18]. Furthermore, Kumar, Srivastav, Wahi, Singh, and Singh [19] found that 6 months of a bacosides-enriched standardised extract of Brahmi (BESEB-CDRI 08; n = 41) significantly improved anxiety, sleep abnormality, and wellbeing (all measured on a VAS) *cf.* placebo (n = 13) in a randomised, double-blind, placebo-controlled cross-over trial.

Other work has produced inconsistent results. For example, 450 mg/day of standardised Brahmi extract (Bacomind®) for 12 weeks (n = 72, aged 35–60 years) showed no improvement in cognition (Rey Auditory Verbal Learning Task [RAVLT], Inspection Time task, Rapid Visual Information Processing [RVIP] Test, and Stroop task) and a trend towards lower state anxiety measured on the STAI for active compared to placebo in a randomised, double-blind, placebo-controlled study [20]. It is possible that discrepancies arise from the cohort tested (i.e., mostly young healthy, non-clinical adults), especially in light of a recent review of randomised controlled trials suggesting that there is evidence for Brahmi as an anxiolytic for people with cognitive decline [21].

4.2.4 Conclusion

The cognitive-enhancing properties of Brahmi have been demonstrated in a wide range of studies and confirmed in systematic reviews, with a meta-analysis on nine randomised controlled trials showing improved executive function and increased attentional processing speed [22], and another meta-analysis on six trials showing that Brahmi improves free recall memory [23]. However, regarding the putative anxiolytic effects of Brahmi, further work is needed to identify target cohorts that may be responsive to these effects, as well as the most effective doses for acute and chronic administration.

4.3 Ginkgo (*Ginkgo biloba*)

4.3.1 Overview

Ginkgo biloba (known as ginkgo) is the only surviving species of the plant division Ginkgophyta, an unusual nonflowering tree that can be traced back over 250 million years [24]. Although native to China, ginkgo is widely cultivated, and has been used since early human history as both a food and a traditional medicine. Ginkgo is thought to reduce the effects of ageing by buffering against oxidative stress. Both the ginkgo leaf and seed have been used in traditional medicine; however, modern research typically focuses on a standardised ginkgo extract: EGb 761.

4.3.2 Mechanisms of Action

4.3.2.1 Constituents

Ginkgo's active constituents are powerful antioxidants. Flavonoids account for 24 % (primarily kaempferol, quercetin, and isorhamnetin) and terpenoids 6 % (ginkgolides A, B, C, and J, and bilobalide) of the standardised EGb 761 extract [25]. Mechanisms of action are thought to include antioxidant, neurotransmitter (increased norepinephrine turnover) and receptor density modulation (increased muscarinic ACh and serotonin receptor density), inhibition of platelet aggregation/anti-platelet activation (particularly ginkgolide B) [26], inhibition of lipid modulation, and delay of hypoxic glycolysis [27]. Anxiolytic effects could result from flavonoid-related serotonin modulation (specifically quercetin), increasing synaptic 5-HT availability [28], and increased brain-derived neurotrophic factor (BDNF) expression [29].

4.3.3 Evidence of Efficacy

4.3.3.1 Preclinical

Animal studies have shown ginkgo to act as a cognitive anxiolytic by facilitating behavioural adaptation, decreasing corticosterone, and inducing anxiolytic activity [30]. For example, Belviranli and Okudan [31] reported improved cognition (increased platform crossings in the Morris water maze), decreased oxidative stress, and increased BDNF in aged female rats following 30 days of ginkgo extract. Ward et al. [32] found that 100 mg/kg/day of standardised ginkgo extract (EGb 761) for 82 days reduced the anxiety that is observed after cold water exposure in male mice after completing Morris water maze tasks. An acute study showed that doses of 50 and 100 mg/kg of Indian origin ginkgo decreased serotonin, and increased norepinephrine and dopamine in rat brains [33].

4.3.3.2 Clinical

Clinical studies examining the chronic cognitive-enhancing anxiolytic properties of ginkgo have shown mixed results. Treatment for 1 week with 120 mg/day standardised ginkgo extract (LI 1370; n = 15) did not affect menopausal symptoms, aggression, or sleepiness, but did improve non-verbal memory, executive function and sustained attention in postmenopausal women (aged 53–65 years), compared to placebo (n = 16) [34]. However, administration of either 240 mg or 480 mg doses of EGb 761 ginkgo extract for 4 weeks significantly reduced Hamilton Rating Scale for Anxiety (HAM-A) scores compared to placebo in participants diagnosed with GAD (n = 82) or adjustment disorder with anxious mood (n = 25) using Diagnostic and Statistical Manual III - Revised (DSM-III-R) criteria in a double-blind, randomised, placebo-controlled trial [35].

Chronic ginkgo administration has also been widely studied as a possible treatment for dementia. For example, participants with mild cognitive impairment (MCI) and neuropsychiatric symptoms (n = 160) receiving 240 mg of EGb 761 standardised ginkgo extract for 24 weeks showed significant improvements in state anxiety (STAI), cognition (attention and executive function), and informants' global impression of change compared to placebo in a randomised, double-blind, placebo-controlled trial [36]. A review found that chronic administration of EGb 761 standardised ginkgo extract improved cognitive impairment due to depression or dementia (with a focus on behavioural and psychological symptoms) [37]. That study also reported improved activities of daily living, and concluded that ginkgo might be useful for people living with dementia who have difficulties with behavioural and psychological symptoms (e.g., agitation and negative mood). However, a large (n = 2487) 5-year randomised, double-blind, placebo-controlled trial of 120 mg/day of EGb 761 standardised ginkgo extract did not show any reduction in risk of progression to Alzheimer's disease (AD) for older adults with memory complaints [38]. Similarly, meta-analyses have shown mixed results, with many concluding that ginkgo does not significantly improve cognition in people with dementia or MCI [39] and that ginkgo is not effective for the treatment of cognition and negative mood in patients with schizophrenia [40]. This pattern of results differs to observations from randomised trials in healthy adults, suggesting that ginkgo may not be as effective as a cognitive enhancer or anxiolytic for cohorts with a high degree of neuroinflammation and oxidative stress.

4.3.4 Conclusion

These inconsistencies are largely due to a lack of fully powered, rigorously conducted randomised controlled trials with a low risk of bias. There is also a similar consensus in the animal literature, with many reviews concluding that there is a need for further work examining the efficacy of ginkgo as a cognitive anxiolytic.

4.4 Lemon Balm (*Melissa officinalis*)

4.4.1 Overview

Melissa officinalis, commonly known as lemon balm, is part of the mint (*Lamiaceae*) family and is naturalised across the world. It is commonly used to flavour food and drinks (e.g., herbal tea), as an essential oil in aromatherapy, as a mosquito repellent (*M. officinalis* Citronella), and is part of several traditional medicine systems (e.g., settling gastrointestinal tract upsets, reducing heart palpitations, mild antibacterial properties, and both anxiolytic and cognitive-enhancing effects). Its cognitive anxiolytic properties have been observed after oral (capsule, coated tablet, beverage, yoghurt drink, and confectionary bar) and topical administration [41]. Studies with oral administration often use a standardised lemon balm extract such as Cyracos®.

4.4.2 Mechanisms of Action

Lemon balm contains a range of bioactive components including flavonoids (e.g., luteolin), phenolic acids (e.g., rosmarinic acid, caffeic acid, and chlorogenic acids), tanins, and triterpenic acids. Lemon balm extract has been shown to bind to both nicotinic and muscarinic cholinergic receptors [42, 43], and interact with GABA-A receptors [44], producing anxiolytic effects. In vitro work has shown that lemon balm extract binds to muscarinic M1 receptors [45]; however, any binding to other receptor subtypes that may influence cognition (e.g., nicotinic $\alpha 4\beta 2$ and $\alpha 7$ and muscarinic M2 and M4 receptors) is largely unknown [46]. Other work has suggested that lemon balm may modulate serotonergic neurotransmission, but is yet to be corroborated [47].

4.4.3 Evidence of Efficacy

4.4.3.1 Preclinical

Animal work examining the anxiolytic effects of lemon balm extract has produced relatively consistent results. Chronic administration (15 days) of lemon balm extract (Cyracos®) resulted in a dose-dependent reduction in anxiety-like reactivity in mice during an elevated plus maze task, but had no effect in an open field task [48]. Three weeks administration of lemon balm increased cell proliferation and GABA, and decreased serum corticosterone levels in mice [49]. Taiwo et al. [50] found comparable anxiolytic effects of lemon balm to diazepam in rats after acute and sub-acute dosing. However, Raines et al. [51] suggested that luteolin, a lemon balm flavonoid, does not exert anxiolytic effects via modulation of GABA-A receptors, but rather affects motor movements and locomotion, suggesting that perhaps other active constituents are binding to GABA-A receptors.

4.4.3.2 Acute Studies in Non-clinical Adults

Randomised controlled trials have shown modest improvements in cognition and reductions in anxiety in healthy adults. Kennedy et al. [52] found that single doses of lemon balm extract (300, 600, 900 mg) improved attentional accuracy and calmness, but also exerted a sedative effect resulting in reduced alertness, secondary memory, and working memory in a randomised, double-blind, placebo-controlled, cross-over study ($n = 20$). A similar single dose (300 and 600 mg) study ($n = 18$) showed that lemon balm ameliorated negative mood from a laboratory-induced stress task, and increased mathematical processing speed [53]. Further, Scholey et al. [41] showed that confectionary bars containing 0.6 g of lemon balm extract significantly improved memory in a double-blind, placebo-controlled, cross-over study in healthy young adults ($n = 25$).

4.4.3.3 Research in Clinical Cohorts

There is some preliminary evidence on the efficacy of lemon balm in improving clinical anxiety. A pilot, open-label study on individuals who met DSM-IV-TR criteria for a primary diagnosis of anxiety disorders and sleep disturbances ($n = 20$) (specific disorders not specified) demonstrated that 15 days of standardised lemon balm extract (Cyracos®) reduced anxiety manifestations, anxiety-associated symptoms, and insomnia as rated on Free Rating Scale for Anxiety (FRSA) and the Clinical Global Impression-Improvement (CGI-I) scale [54]. Results should be interpreted with caution, however, due to the lack of comparison with a placebo.

Due to its cholinergic binding properties, lemon balm has been examined as a potential treatment for the cognitive deficits in AD. Ballard et al. [55] found that lemon balm essential oil aromatherapy reduced agitation and social withdrawal, and increased engagement in constructive activities in patients with severe dementia ($n = 72$), compared to placebo. A 16-week double-blind placebo-controlled trial in participants with mild to moderate AD ($n = 42$) evidenced significantly improved cognitive function and reduced agitation after 60 drops/day of lemon balm extract compared to placebo [56]. A more recent study compared 4 weeks ($n = 94$) administration of lemon balm aromatherapy to donepezil and placebo in participants with probable or possible AD [57]. Interestingly, behavioural and psychological symptoms of AD, including agitation, decreased across all three groups (Pittsburgh Agitation Scale [PAS] scores), suggesting that lemon balm is not superior to placebo or donepezil. The authors concluded that improvement across the groups was most likely due to non-specific benefits of interaction and touch.

4.4.4 Conclusion

There are some promising findings on the efficacy of lemon balm as a cognitive anxiolytic from animal studies and randomised controlled trials involving healthy adults. Further work is required to ascertain whether it has efficacy in a clinical setting, particularly for anxiety disorders. Findings on the cognitive-enhancing properties of lemon balm in people living with dementia also require replication. Further in vitro work would assist in identifying lemon balm's receptor binding sites and specific mechanisms of action.

4.5 Tea (*Camellia sinensis*)

4.5.1 Overview

The leaves and buds of *Camellia sinesis* are used to produce the popular beverage, tea, including green, black, oolong, white, and yellow tea varieties. *Camellia sinesis* is part of the Theaceae family of flowering plants, and the two major varieties grown are *Camellia sinesis* var. *sinesis* (Chinese teas) and *Camellia sinesis* var. *assamica* (Indian Assam teas). Tea is cultivated across the world and has been consumed throughout human history for a variety of health, social, and cultural reasons, and has been used in traditional medicine systems including Chinese herbal medicine. Data from epidemiological studies suggest that drinking tea (mostly green tea) may boost cognition, helping to protect the brain against ageing [58–60], and reduce psychological distress [61] (Table 4.1).

4.5.2 Mechanisms of Action

4.5.2.1 Constituents

The primary bioactive constituents of tea are polyphenols, amino acids, and caffeine [62]. Between 30 and 42 % of the dry weight of green tea is formed from catechins; caffeine and L-theanine (amino acid) respectively account for around 2 to 5 % and 3 %. Its chief catechin polyphenol, epigallocatechin gallate (EGCG), contributes 50 to 80 % of total catechins [63], and has neuroprotective effects due to its antioxidant action, suppressing inflammatory processes and inhibiting cell proliferation [64]. Other prominent catechins include epigallocatechin (EGC), epicatechin gallate (ECG), and epicatechin (EC), although these are present in smaller quantities. L-theanine is a non-protein amino acid analogue of γ-N-ethyl-L-glutamine, and has been shown to bind to AMPA (α-amino-3-hydroxy-5-methyl-4-isoxazolepropionic acid), *N*-Methyl-D-aspartate (NMDA), group I metabotropic glutamate, and kainate receptors, inhibiting glutamate reuptake and potentiating GABA, dopamine, and serotonin [65–67]. L-theanine is thought to have anxiolytic properties due to potentiation of GABA [68], the primary inhibitory neurotransmitter in the brain. Caffeine inhibits adenosine (A1 and A2a) receptors, increasing dopamine transmission and ACh, resulting in increased arousal and enhanced cognition [69]. These three constituents are thought to interact, resulting in the overall cognitive-enhancing and anxiolytic effects of tea, with some evidence that L-Theanine inhibits caffeine's stimulatory effects [70].

Table 4.1 List of herbal medicines used as cognitive anxiolytics, typical dosage, active constituents, summary of evidence, potential adverse effects, potential clinical use, and clinical advice

Herbal medicine	Dosage	Major/active constituents	Key evidence	Potential adverse effects	Potential clinical use	Clinical advice
Brahmi (*Bacopa monnieri*)	Acute: 320 mg or 640 mg of Brahmi extract Chronic: 300 mg/d or 450 mg/d of Brahmi extract for 12 weeks or 6 months	Bacosides A and B	Some positive Randomised Controlled Trials (RCTs) and two meta-analyses showing significant reductions in trait anxiety and improvements in cognitive function (executive function, processing speed, free recall) versus placebo	No adverse reactions found in studies	Non-clinical stress or anxiety, anxiety-induced insomnia, anxiety associated with cognitive decline. Further research needed on individuals with clinical anxiety disorders Some suggestion it may have equivalent effects to benzodiazepines and therefore may be a useful alternative to these	Generally safe, though currently no data on potential interactions with psychotropic medications. Use with care
Ginkgo (*Ginkgo biloba*)	Standardised ginkgo extract: EGb 761 240 mg/d or 480 mg/d for 4 weeks or 24 weeks	Flavonoids (kaempferol, quercetin, and isorhamnetin) Terpenoids (ginkgolides A, B, C, J, and bilobalide)	Some positive RCTs for anxiety and cognitive function, though several meta-analyses have concluded null effects	No adverse reactions found in studies	GAD, anxiety associated with adjustment disorder, anxiety associated with mild cognitive impairment (MCI)	Generally safe, though currently no data on potential interactions with psychotropic medications. Can lead to excessive bleeding and bruising when used with antiplatelet aggregators. Has known effects on neurotransmitters (particularly serotonin, norepinephrine, and dopamine), therefore, use with care

(continued)

Table 4.1 (continued)

Herbal medicine	Dosage	Major/active constituents	Key evidence	Potential adverse effects	Potential clinical use	Clinical advice
Lemon balm (*Melissa officinalis*)	Acute: 300, 600, or 900 mg of lemon balm extract Chronic: 60 drops/d of lemon balm extract for 16 weeks; standardised lemon balm extract (Cyracos®) for 15 days	Flavonoids (e.g., luteolin). Phenolic acids (e.g., rosmarinic acid, caffeic acid, and chlorogenic acids). Tanins. Triterpenic acids	Some positive RCTs for anxiety and cognitive function (attention, processing speed, memory)	No adverse reactions found in studies; commonly added to food as flavouring or consumed as a tea	Mild-to-moderate clinical anxiety (DMS-IV-TR), insomnia, agitation, and anxiety associated with dementia (including AD). Some suggestion it may have equivalent effects to benzodiazepines and therefore may be a useful alternative to these	Generally safe and widely consumed
Tea (*Camellia sinensis*)	Acute: 75 mg caffeine ±50 mg L-theanine. Chronic: 8 weeks of 400 mg/day L-theanine	Polyphenols (e.g., catechins). Amino acids (e.g., L-theanine). Caffeine	Some positive RCTs on cognitive function (alertness, attentional switching) and anxiety for constituents of tea (particularly L-theanine + caffeine), however, overall meta-analyses have failed to confirm the cognitive anxiolytic effects	No adverse reactions found in studies; commonly consumed as a drink	Non-clinical stress, tension, or anxiety, anxiety associated with schizophrenia or schizoaffective disorder. Further research needed on individuals with clinical anxiety disorders. The cognitive anxiolytic effects are currently questionable and further research is needed prior to formal recommendations. It is also currently unclear which combination of L-theanine and caffeine is ideal	Generally safe and widely consumed

Sage (*Salvia* spp.)	Acute: 25 μL or 50 μL (essential oil) of *S. lavandulaefolia* OR 300 mg or 600 mg (dried leaf) of *S. officinalis* Chronic: 6 weeks oral administration (50 μL essential oil up to 3 times per day) of *S. lavandulaefolia* OR 16 weeks oral administration of 60 drops per day of 1:1 plant extract (i.e., 1 kg leaf: 1 L 45 % alcohol) of *S. officinalis*	Terpenoids (e.g., 1,8-cineole, α- and β-pinene, camphor, bornyl acetate, 3-carene)	Pre-clinical research and traditional use suggest potential anxiolytic effects; two positive RCTs in humans demonstrating acute anxiolytic effects RCTs in MCI and AD suggest cognitive-enhancing effects	No adverse reactions found in studies; commonly used in cooking	Non-clinical stress or anxiety, agitation and anxiety associated with cognitive decline (MCI, AD). Further research needed on individuals with clinical anxiety disorders	Generally safe and widely consumed
Rosemary (*Rosmarinus officinalis*)	Acute: aromatherapy essential oil inhalation (3–4 drops on cotton wool) or massage (20 min)	Rosmarinic acid Terpenoids (e.g., 1,8-cineole, α-pinene, camphor)	A systematic review suggests positive anxiolytic effects, though the unique effects of rosemary versus aromatherapy in general (including lavender) remains unclear Some positive RCTs indicate acute improvements in cognitive function (e.g., alertness, memory)	No adverse reactions found in studies; commonly used in cooking and aromatherapy	Non-clinical stress or anxiety, test anxiety, anxiety associated with medical conditions or an adjustment disorder. Further research needed on individuals with clinical anxiety disorders Some suggestion in pre-clinical research that it may have equivalent effects to benzodiazepines and therefore may be a useful alternative to these	Generally safe and widely consumed

4.5.3 Evidence of Efficacy

4.5.3.1 Preclinical

Animal studies have demonstrated effects of green tea extract and its individual constituents on cognition and anxiety. Work on green tea extract has demonstrated effects after both chronic and acute administration. Improvements in motor coordination (Morris water maze, rota rod test, locomotor activity measured with actophotometer, and negative geotaxis measured with mid-air righting) and reduced anxiety (elevated plus maze, open field test) in valproic acid induced oxidative stress model mice were seen after 300 mg/kg of green tea extract [71]. In addition, enhanced learning and memory in aged rats were observed after 8 weeks of 0.5 % green tea extract, measured by elevated plus maze and passive avoidance tests [72]. Other acute research on individual constituents showed that standardised EGCG extract (10 mg/kg) reduced cognitive dysfunction and improved positive mood in Parkinson's disease model rats [73], and that 100 μml/20 g of EGCG resulted in amnestic and anxiolytic effects on behaviour in mice in elevated plus maze test [74]. However, Stringer, Abeysekera, Dria, Roper, and Goodlett [75] did not show cognitive improvement in Down syndrome model mice following chronic administration of EGCG (~20 mg/kg/day) for 3 or 7 weeks. Heese et al. [68] found that acute 10 mg/kg L-theanine alone did not exert anxiolytic effects; however, when combined with midazolam, a synergistic/additive effect occurred, resulting in decreased anxiety and motor movements on the elevated plus maze. L-theanine has also been shown to reduce opioid withdrawal signs in rhesus monkeys (e.g., fighting), and produce anxiolytic effects in mice without affecting motor behaviour [70].

4.5.3.2 Clinical

Work examining the combined and separate effects of acute L-theanine and caffeine on human cognition and mood has demonstrated that L-theanine suppresses the stimulatory effect of caffeine. For example, a study on the acute effects of caffeine and L-theanine in habitual (n = 12) and non-habitual (n = 12) caffeine drinkers demonstrated that 75 mg caffeine alone improved attention and positive mood (VAS), reduced oxygenated haemoglobin, and increased deoxygenated haemoglobin [76]. When 75 mg caffeine and 50 mg L-theanine were combined, increased deoxygenated haemoglobin was still apparent; however, this was somewhat attenuated compared to caffeine alone. Those authors concluded that caffeine and L-theanine interact, and the presence of L-theanine results in the attenuation of the vasoconstrictive and behavioural effects of caffeine. Further research is required to identify which constituent contributes to the positive effects on mood. Another study (n = 48) showed that acute dosing of caffeine (250 mg) increased alertness, jitteriness, and blood pressure, but when combined with 200 mg L-theanine, caffeine's effect on blood pressure was attenuated; L-theanine alone slowed reaction times on a visual probe task [77]. Importantly, Camfield et al. [78] conducted a meta-analysis on 11 randomised placebo-controlled trials to determine the acute effects of EGCG, L-Theanine, and caffeine. Combined caffeine and L-theanine was found to improve cognition (alertness and attentional switching accuracy); however, a subsequent analysis showed a trend towards an enhanced effect for caffeine compared to L-theanine.

Other research utilising L-theanine alone has demonstrated anxiolytic effects. A randomised controlled trial ($n = 60$) on 8 weeks of 400 mg/day L-theanine administration significantly reduced anxiety and positive psychopathology scores (on the Positive and Negative Affect Schedule [PANAS]) in participants with a DSM-IV diagnosis of schizophrenia or schizoaffective disorder [79]. In relation to acute studies, Lu et al. [65] demonstrated that 200 mg L-theanine exerts calming effects under resting conditions (measured on visual analogue mood scale [VAMS]), however does not demonstrate anxiolytic effects under increased anxiety conditions ($n = 16$). Further, a recent study ($n = 34$) on the effects of an L-theanine-based nutrient drink (197 mg L-theanine) on responses to a cognitive stressor demonstrated a reduced salivary cortisol response and increased magnetoencephalogram (MEG) alpha activity (indicating decreased cortical arousal) following treatment, *cf.* placebo, for individuals higher in trait anxiety (STAI) [80]. Other work has shown that 200 mg L-theanine significantly attenuates task-related blood-pressure increases in labile individuals ($n = 14$), and reduced tension-anxiety scores measured on the Profile of Mood States (POMS) [81]. In the meta-analysis by Camfield et al. [78], no overall acute effects on anxiety were found in the first two hours post-dose, as measured by the STAI. However, isolated studies [77, 82] that were included in the review did report anxiolytic effects for 200 mg L-theanine in comparison to placebo (with standardised mean differences [SMDs] from 0.42 to 0.84).

The flavonoid EGCG has received less attention in human trials. A double-blind, placebo-controlled, cross-over design study ($n = 31$) reported that acute administration of 300 mg EGCG increased electroencephalogram (EEG) alpha, beta, and theta activity, increased self-reported calmness, and reduced self-reported stress [83]. Wightman, Haskell, Forster, Veasey, and Kennedy [84] found that 135 mg acute administration of EGCG reduced heart rate, oxygenated and total haemoglobin in the frontal cortex, but did not affect cognitive performance or mood ($n = 27$). An fMRI study ($n = 12$) found an acute dose-dependent effect of green tea extract in a milk whey based soft drink (0.05 % extract/250 ml or 500 ml) on increased activation in the dorso-lateral prefrontal cortex *cf.* controls, in a working memory task [85].

4.5.4 Conclusion

A small number of human trials have focused on the combined and separate effects of EGCG, L-theanine, and caffeine on cognition and anxiety, and reported findings consistent with anecdotal reasons for tea consumption. This work has demonstrated that the active constituents of tea have cognitive anxiolytic properties, particularly when administered in combination. Further work is needed to elucidate the mechanisms underpinning these combined/synergistic effects.

4.6 Sage (*Salvia spp.*)

4.6.1 Overview

Commonly referred to as Sage, the *Salvia* genus (e.g., *S. officinalis*, *S. lavandulaefolia*, and *S. elegans*) belongs to the mint (*Lamiaceae*) family and includes almost 1000 species from across the world. Common uses include cooking or traditional medicinal herbs, ornamental plants, and occasionally religious ceremonies. More recent clinical applications of sage typically take the form of a standardised essential oil extract in combination with an inactive agent (e.g., sunflower oil) or dried plant extract in an alcohol solution, for oral administration [42, 86].

4.6.2 Mechanisms of Action

4.6.2.1 Constituents

The main active constituents of sage, relevant to anxiety, are the class of terpenoids (e.g., 1,8-cineole, α- and β-pinene, camphor, bornyl acetate, 3-carene), which are AChE and butyrylcholinesterase (BuChE) inhibitors [42]. Even very low concentrations of sage (*S. officinalis* or *S. lavandulaefolia*) have demonstrated anti-AChE activity both in vitro [87, 88] and in vivo [89], and anti-BuChE activity in vitro [90]. These, and other constituents (e.g., carvacrol, luteolin, and rosmarinic acid), have also reliably demonstrated antioxidant, anti-inflammatory, and oestrogenic activities in vivo [91].

4.6.3 Evidence of Efficacy

4.6.3.1 Anxiety

Despite traditional uses, relatively few empirical studies have investigated the anxiolytic properties of sage in humans. The pre-clinical research on *S. elegans* [92, 93], *S. leriifolia* [94], *S. reuterana* [95], and *S. miltiorrhiza* [96] has demonstrated clinically significant anxiolytic effects using mouse and rat models and the elevated plus maze. In healthy (non-clinical) humans, one randomised, placebo-controlled, double-blind, balanced, cross-over design study in young adults ($n = 24$; $M_{age} = 23.2$ years) demonstrated significant increases in subjective feelings of 'calmness' (Bond-Lader mood scale) following a single dose (25 μL or 50 μL essential oil) of *S. lavandulaefolia* [97]. A similarly designed study in non-clinical young adults ($n = 30$; $M_{age} = 24.4$ years) demonstrated acute (up to, but not beyond 20 min) anxiolytic effects (Bond-Lader mood scale, STAI-state) of a single dose (300 mg or 600 mg dried leaf) of *S. officinalis* [98], though a more recent study with a similar design failed to find any anxiolytic effects of *S. lavandulaefolia* [99].

4.6.3.2 Cognitive Function

In pre-clinical research, *S. officinalis* increased memory retention in rats in a passive avoidance learning paradigm [100]. In healthy humans, randomised, placebo-controlled, double-blind, balanced, cross-over design studies in young (approx. M_{age} = 23–24 years) [97–99, 101] and older (n = 20; M_{age} = 73.0 years) [102] adults have demonstrated significant improvements in measures of attention, alertness, processing speed, and memory (including immediate and delayed word recall, picture recognition, and speed of memory) from a single dose of either *S. lavandulaefolia* or *S. officinalis*. Interestingly, to date the only clinical trials of sage have investigated their efficacy for use in dementia populations, including individuals with MCI and AD. One pilot open-label study demonstrated significant improvements in attention following 6-week oral administration (50 μL essential oil up to 3 times per day) of *S. lavandulaefolia* to individuals (n = 11; aged 76–95 years) with mild to moderate AD [91]. Similarly, a parallel group, placebo-controlled, double-blind clinical trial demonstrated significant improvements in overall cognitive function (including measures of attention, memory, orientation, and problem-solving) following 16-week oral administration of 60 drops per day of 1:1 plant extract (i.e., 1 kg leaf: 1 L 45 % alcohol) of *S. officinalis* to individuals (n = 42; aged 65–80 years) with mild to moderate AD [103]. This study also found a potential ad hoc side effect of reduced agitation in comparison to the placebo group, suggesting potential anxiolytic effects. However, one pre-clinical study demonstrated impairments to cognitive function (despite anxiolytic effects) following administration of *S. elegans* [93].

4.6.4 Conclusion

Preliminary findings suggest promising effects after oral administration of sage (particularly *S. officinalis* or *S. lavandulaefolia*) as a cognitive enhancer in individuals with AD and an anxiolytic in healthy, non-clinical individuals. However, to date no studies have investigated the effects of sage as a cognitive anxiolytic in individuals with a clinical anxiety disorder. Nor have studies investigated the long-term effects of sage on cognitive function. Further research is needed.

4.7 Rosemary (*Rosmarinus officinalis*)

4.7.1 Overview

Commonly referred to as Rosemary, *Rosmarinus officinalis* is also a member of the mint (*Lamiaceae*) family. Recent clinical applications of rosemary involve aromatherapy of the essential oil via the skin (massage) or olfactory system (inhalation).

4.7.2 Mechanisms of Action

4.7.2.1 Constituents

The main active constituents of rosemary relevant to anxiety are the phenolic acid rosmarinic acid and the terpenoids 1,8-cineole, α-pinene, and camphor, which have been shown to increase ACh and produce differential effects on AChE [104, 105]. Inhalation and oral administration of rosemary oil resulted in increases in blood levels of 1,8-cineole in mice [106]. Intragastric administration of either *R. officinalis* plant extract or rosmarinic acid resulted in an inhibition of AChE but an increase in BuChE activity in the hippocampus and frontal cortex of rats [107].

4.7.3 Evidence of Efficacy

4.7.3.1 Cognitive Function

In pre-clinical research, intragastric administration of *R. officinalis* extract improved long-term memory and reversed chemically induced (scopolamine) memory impairment in rats [107]. In healthy humans, skin application of 1,8-cineole was associated with faster reaction time on a vigilance task than (±)-linalool [108]. Similarly, a large ($n = 144$) randomised, parallel-group study of healthy young adults demonstrated significantly increased alertness and higher performance on multiple memory tests (including immediate and delayed word recall, word and picture recognition, and working memory) following acute administration of rosemary aromatherapy inhalation compared to either the lavender or control groups [109]. Acute administration of rosemary aromatherapy inhalation was also associated with a significant decrease in frontal EEG alpha power (suggesting increased alertness) compared to lavender aromatherapy [110].

4.7.3.2 Anxiety

In pre-clinical research, rosemary oils have exhibited clinically significant anxiolytic effects using rodent models and the elevated plus maze [see 111 for systematic review]. More specifically, either long-term oral [112] or acute intraperitoneal [113] administration of *R. officinalis* plant extract have demonstrated anxiolytic effects in mice using the elevated plus maze (and equivalence to diazepam) [113]. In healthy (non-clinical) humans ($n = 40$), acute aromatherapy inhalation of rosemary essential oil was associated with significantly lower test anxiety (test anxiety inventory [TAI]) and heart rate than the control (no aromatherapy) condition [114]. A quasi-experimental, control group, pretest-posttest design study of healthy older adults (65–85 years; $n = 36$) demonstrated significantly greater reduction in state anxiety (STAI) following tri-weekly, 20 min aromatherapy massage of rosemary (with lavender, chamomile, and lemon, in an essential oil diluted with jojoba) for a total of 6 weeks, than those who received no intervention [115]. A systematic review of 16 randomised controlled trials confirmed that aromatherapy (typically rosemary and/or lavender) had significant anxiolytic effects in individuals with anxiety symptoms [e.g., medical patients; 116]. However, relatively few studies have investigated the unique anxiolytic effects of rosemary as compared to another aromatherapy essential oil such as lavender. One study suggested that acute administration of lavender aromatherapy inhalation but not rosemary has significant anxiolytic effects [117], whereas other work has demonstrated comparable anxiolytic effects of acute administration of rosemary versus lavender [110].

4.7.4 Conclusion

Preliminary findings suggest promising effects of rosemary aromatherapy (via massage or inhalation) as an anxiolytic in both healthy individuals and those experiencing clinical levels of anxiety. Furthermore, there is support for rosemary as a cognitive enhancer. However, a major limitation of the literature is the absence of a standardised practice regarding dosage and/or content ratio of aromatherapy oils. Thus, it is difficult to differentiate the unique effects of rosemary versus other essential oils (particularly lavender). There is also potential bias in aromatherapy research due to problems with blinding, considering the difficulty involved in administering an equivalent placebo treatment. Similarly, there are no apparent standardised practices surrounding the massage protocol. As such, the unique effects or additional benefits of aromatherapy massage versus touch massage (i.e., without essential oils) versus other types of massage remain unclear [see 118 for recent reviews of the anxiolytic benefits of massage therapy, 119, 120]. Further research is warranted.

4.8 Clinical Considerations and Future Directions

One of the difficulties in assessing the cognitive anxiolytic efficacy of herbal medicines is the use of standardised extracts. Furthermore, many traditional medicinal systems use multi-herb formulas, which may have synergistic effects (e.g., increasing bioavailability), making it difficult to separate findings. Further work is needed to ascertain how the various bioactive constituents of these herbs interact to produce both cognitive-enhancing and anxiolytic effects. Currently, little is known regarding the potential interactions of these herbs with existing psychotropic medications such as antidepressants (e.g., SSRIs, SNRIs, and tricyclics), anxiolytics (e.g., benzodiazepines), or antipsychotics, particularly atypical antipsychotics (e.g., quetiapine, olanzapine, risperidone, and aripiprazole) which are commonly prescribed for insomnia and sleep-related difficulties (though there is limited evidence to support their efficacy in such cases) [see 121 for discussion]. While there is some suggestion that certain herbs such as Brahmi, lemon balm, and rosemary may provide equivalent anxiolytic effects to other benzodiazepines, further research is needed.

Future studies would also benefit from utilising samples with clinical anxiety disorders. Typically, clinical samples have a larger range and distribution of symptoms, and these tend to be more severe and chronic in nature. Investigating the effects of herbal medicines in these samples will provide a better representation of their potential for cognitive anxiolytic effects. Similarly, long-term follow-up studies will better inform the capacity these herbs have for exerting enduring changes on anxiety levels.

While further research is needed, there is an increasing body of evidence in support of the cognitive anxiolytic effects of certain herbal medicines, particularly as there are currently no suggestions of significant negative side effects or contraindications associated with those discussed in this chapter. Lemon balm (*M. officinalis*), tea (*Camellia sinensis*), and sage (*Salvia* spp.) appear the most promising of those outlined here.

Anxiety disorders such as GAD and PD are characterised by somatic symptoms including muscle tension, restlessness, heart palpitations, chest pain, or difficulty breathing [122] which may benefit from the immediate physiological effects of anxiolytics. Anxiety disorders are also associated with clinical symptoms such as difficulties with concentration and fatigue [122] and cognitive deficits such as poor attention and memory [1–4], which may be specifically ameliorated by cognitive anxiolytics. However, beyond these direct putative effects, there are strong clinical arguments for the use of cognitive anxiolytics as an adjunct to psychological interventions. Indeed, cognitive behaviour therapy (CBT) is the gold-standard psychological intervention for anxiety disorders, including GAD, PD, and SAD [123–126], and involves using cognitive challenging and restructuring in conjunction with exposure and behavioural experiments to target maintaining factors. In this way, cognitive enhancement may indirectly improve symptoms of anxiety by increasing therapeutic engagement and capacity for comprehension and change.

References

1. Ferreri F, Lapp LK, Peretti CS. Current research on cognitive aspects of anxiety disorders. Curr Opin Psychiatry. 2011;24:49–54.
2. O'Sullivan K, Newman EF. Neuropsychological impairments in panic disorder: a systematic review. J Affect Disord. 2014;167:268–84.
3. O'Toole MS, Pedersen AD. A systematic review of neuropsychological performance in social anxiety disorder. Nord J Psychiatry. 2011;65:147–61.
4. Yang Y et al. Cognitive impairment in generalized anxiety disorder revealed by event-related potential N270. Neuropsychiatr Dis Treat. 2015;11:1405–11.
5. Rickels K, Rynn M. Pharmacotherapy of generalized anxiety disorder. J Clin Psychiatry. 2002;63:9–16.
6. Stewart SA. The effects of benzodiazepines on cognition. J Clin Psychiatry. 2005;66:9–13.
7. Russo A, Borrelli F. Bacopa monniera, a reputed nootropic plant: an overview. Phytomedicine. 2005;12:305–17.
8. Aguiar S, Borowski T. Neuropharmacological review of the nootropic herb Bacopa monnieri. Rejuvenation Res. 2013;16:313–26.
9. Singh HK, Dhawan BN. Neuropsychopharmacological effects of the Ayurvedic nootropic Bacopa monniera Linn (Brahmi). Indian J Pharmacol. 1997;29:359–65.
10. Nathan PJ et al. The acute effects of an extract of Bacopa monniera (Brahmi) on cognitive function in healthy normal subjects. Hum Psychopharmacol. 2001;16:345–51.
11. Downey LA et al. An acute, double-blind, placebo-controlled crossover study of 320 mg and 640 mg doses of a special extract of Bacopa monnieri (CDRI 08) on sustained cognitive performance. Phytother Res. 2013;27:1407–13.

12. Becker RE. Therapy of the cognitive deficit in Alzheimers disease: the cholinergic system. In: Becker RE, Giabcobini E, editors. Cholinergic basis for Alzheimer therapy. Boston: Birkhauser; 1991. p. 1–22.
13. Bhattacharya SK et al. Antioxidant activity of Bacopa monniera in rat frontal cortex, striatum and hippocampus. Phytother Res. 2000;14:174–9.
14. Piyabhan P, Wetchateng T. Neuroprotective effects of Bacopa monnieri (brahmi) on novel object recognition and NMDAR1 immunodensity in the prefrontal cortex, striatum and hippocampus of sub-chronic phencyclidine rat model of schizophrenia. J Med Assoc Thai. 2014;97:S50–6.
15. Vollala VR, Upadhya S, Nayak S. Enhanced dendritic arborization of hippocampal CA3 neurons by Bacopa monniera extract treatment in adult rats. Rom J Morphol Embryol. 2011;52:879–86.
16. Bhattacharya SK, Ghosal S. Anxiolytic activity of a standardized extract of Bacopa monniera: an experimental study. Phytomedicine. 1998;5:77–82.
17. Benson S et al. An acute, double-blind, placebo-controlled cross-over study of 320 mg and 640 mg doses of Bacopa monnieri (CDRI 08) on multitasking stress reactivity and mood. Phytother Res. 2014;28:551–9.
18. Calabrese C et al. Effects of a standardized Bacopa monnieri extract on cognitive performance, anxiety, and depression in the elderly: a randomized, double-blind, placebo-controlled trial. J Altern Complement Med. 2008;14:707–13.
19. Kumar T et al. Randomized control, double blind cross-over study to clinically assess the Rasayana effect of a standardized extract of Brahmi (Bacopa monniera) in adult human volunteers. Int J Pharm Pharm Sci. 2011;3(Suppl 4):263–6.
20. Sathyanarayanan V et al. Brahmi for the better? New findings challenging cognition and anti-anxiety effects of Brahmi (Bacopa monniera) in healthy adults. Psychopharmacology (Berl). 2013;227:299–306.
21. Sarris J, McIntyre E, Camfield DA. Plant-based medicines for anxiety disorders, Part 2: a review of clinical studies with supporting preclinical evidence. CNS Drugs. 2013;27:301–19.
22. Kongkeaw C et al. Meta-analysis of randomized controlled trials on cognitive effects of Bacopa monnieri extract. J Ethnopharmacol. 2014;151:528–35.
23. Pase MP et al. The cognitive-enhancing effects of bacopa monnieri: a systematic review of randomized, controlled human clinical trials. J Altern Complement Med. 2012;18:647–52.
24. Singh B et al. Biology and chemistry of Ginkgo biloba. Fitoterapia. 2008;79:401–18.
25. Christen Y, Maixent JM. What is Ginkgo biloba extract EGb 761? An overview from molecular biology to clinical medicine. Cell Mol Biol. 2002;48(6):601–11.
26. Maclennan KM, Darlington CL, Smith PF. The CNS effects of Ginkgo biloba extracts and ginkgolide B. Prog Neurobiol. 2002;67:235–57.
27. Diamond BJ et al. Ginkgo biloba extract: mechanisms and clinical indications. Arch Phys Med Rehabil. 2000;81:668–78.
28. Domingo MT et al. Inhibition by ginkgolides of the binding of [3H]PAF platelet-activating factor (PAF) to platelet membranes. In: Braquet P, editor. Ginkgolides. Barcelona: JR Prous; 1988. p. 79–84.
29. Hou Y et al. Anti-depressant natural flavonols modulate BDNF and beta amyloid in neurons and hippocampus of double TgAD mice. Neuropharmacology. 2010;58:911–20.
30. DeFeudis FV, Drieu K. "Stress-alleviating" and "vigilance-enhancing" actions of Ginkgo biloba extract (EGb 761). Drug Dev Res. 2004;62:1–25.
31. Belviranli M, Okudan N. The effects of Ginkgo biloba extract on cognitive functions in aged female rats: the role of oxidative stress and brain-derived neurotrophic factor. Behav Brain Res. 2015;278:453–61.
32. Ward CP et al. Ginkgo biloba extract: cognitive enhancer or antistress buffer. Pharmacol Biochem Behav. 2002;72:913–22.
33. Satyan KS et al. Effect of Ginkgolic acid conjugates on the brain monoamines and metabolites in rodents. Biogenic Amines. 1997;13:143–51.

34. Hartley DE et al. Effects on cognition and mood in postmenopausal women of 1-week treatment with Ginkgo biloba. Pharmacol Bioch Behav. 2003;75:711–20.
35. Woelk H et al. Ginkgo biloba special extract EGb 761® in generalized anxiety disorder and adjustment disorder with anxious mood: a randomized, double-blind, placebo-controlled trial. J Psychiatr Res. 2007;41:472–80.
36. Gavrilova SI et al. Efficacy and safety of Ginkgo biloba extract EGb 761® in mild cognitive impairment with neuropsychiatric symptoms: a randomized, placebo-controlled, double-blind, multicenter trial. Int J Geriatr Psychiatry. 2014;29:1087–95.
37. Hoerr R. Behavioural and psychological symptoms of dementia (BPSD): effects of EGb 761®. Pharmacopsychiatry. 2003;36(Suppl 1).
38. Vellas B et al. Long-term use of standardised ginkgo biloba extract for the prevention of Alzheimer's disease (GuidAge): a randomised placebo-controlled trial. Lancet Neurol. 2012;11:851–9.
39. Birks J, Grimley Evans J. Ginkgo biloba for cognitive impairment and dementia. Cochrane Database Syst Rev. 2007;2.
40. Brondino N et al. A systematic review and meta-analysis of ginkgo biloba in neuropsychiatric disorders: from ancient tradition to modern-day medicine. Evid Based Complement Alternat Med. 2013;2013.
41. Scholey A et al. Investigation of a Melissa officinalis special extract on Cognition II: human study – Lemon balm extract administered in confectionary bars. Agro Food Ind Hi-Tech. 2015;26:12–4.
42. Kennedy DO, Scholey AB. The psychopharmacology of European herbs with cognition-enhancing properties. Curr Pharm Des. 2006;12:4613–23.
43. Kennedy DO et al. Modulation of mood and cognitive performance following acute administration of single doses of Melissa officinalis (Lemon balm) with human CNS nicotinic and muscarinic receptor-binding properties. Neuropsychopharmacology. 2003;28:1871–81.
44. Awad R et al. Bioassay-guided fractionation of lemon balm (Melissa officinalis L.) using an in vitro measure of GABA transaminase activity. Phytother Res. 2009;23:1075–81.
45. Buchwald-Werner S, Vazquez I, Röchter S. Investigation of a Melissa officinalis special extract on Cognition I: in vitro study on muscarinic properties. Agro Food Ind Hi-Tech. 2015;26:34–6.
46. Scholey A et al. Anti-stress effects of lemon balm-containing foods. Nutrients. 2014;6:4805–21.
47. Lin SH et al. A medicinal herb, Melissa officinalis L. ameliorates depressive-like behavior of rats in the forced swimming test via regulating the serotonergic neurotransmitter. J Ethnopharmacol. 2015;175:266–72.
48. Ibarra A et al. Effects of chronic administration of Melissa officinalis L. extract on anxiety-like reactivity and on circadian and exploratory activities in mice. Phytomedicine. 2010;17:397–403.
49. Yoo DY et al. Effects of Melissa officinalis L. (Lemon Balm) extract on neurogenesis associated with serum corticosterone and GABA in the mouse dentate gyrus. Neurochem Res. 2011;36:250–7.
50. Taiwo AE et al. Anxiolytic and antidepressant-like effects of Melissa officinalis (lemon balm) extract in rats: influence of administration and gender. Indian J Pharmacol. 2012;44:189–92.
51. Raines T et al. Investigation of the anxiolytic effects of luteolin, a lemon balm flavonoid in the male Sprague-Dawley rat. AANA J. 2009;77:33–6.
52. Kennedy DO et al. Modulation of mood and cognitive performance following acute administration of Melissa officinalis (lemon balm). Pharmacol Biochem Behav. 2002;72:953–64.
53. Kennedy DO, Little W, Scholey AB. Attenuation of laboratory-induced stress in humans after acute administration of Melissa officinalis (lemon balm). Psychosom Med. 2004;66:607–13.
54. Cases J et al. Pilot trial of Melissa officinalis L. leaf extract in the treatment of volunteers suffering from mild-to-moderate anxiety disorders and sleep disturbances. Med J Nutrition Metab. 2011;4:211–8.

55. Ballard CG et al. Aromatherapy as a safe and effective treatment for the management of agitation in severe dementia: the results of a double-blind, placebo-controlled trial with Melissa. J Clin Psychiatry. 2002;63:553–8.
56. Akhondzadeh S et al. Melissa officinalis extract in the treatment of patients with mild to moderate Alzheimer's disease: a double blind, randomised, placebo controlled trial. J Neurol Neurosur Psychiatry. 2003;74:863–6.
57. Burns A et al. A double-blind placebo-controlled randomized trial of melissa officinalis oil and donepezil for the treatment of agitation in Alzheimer's disease. Dement Geriatr Cogn Disord. 2011;31:158–64.
58. Feng L et al. Cognitive function and tea consumption in community dwelling older Chinese in Singapore. J Nutr Health Aging. 2010;14:433–8.
59. Kuriyama S et al. Green tea consumption and cognitive function: a cross-sectional study from the Tsurugaya Project 1. Am J Clin Nutr. 2006;83:355–61.
60. Ng TP et al. Tea consumption and cognitive impairment and decline in older Chinese adults. Am J Clin Nutr. 2008;88:224–31.
61. Hozawa A et al. Green tea consumption is associated with lower psychological distress in a general population: the Ohsaki Cohort 2006 Study. Am J Clin Nutr. 2009;90:1390–6.
62. Sharangi AB. Medicinal and therapeutic potentialities of tea (Camellia sinensis L.) – a review. Food Res Int. 2009;42:529–35.
63. Graham HN. Green tea composition, consumption, and polyphenol chemistry. Prev Med. 1992;21:334–50.
64. Singh BN, Shankar S, Srivastava RK. Green tea catechin, epigallocatechin-3-gallate (EGCG): mechanisms, perspectives and clinical applications. Biochem Pharmacol. 2011;82:1807–21.
65. Lu K et al. The acute effects of L-theanine in comparison with alprazolam on anticipatory anxiety in humans. Hum Psychopharmacol. 2004;19:457–65.
66. Yokogoshi H et al. Effect of theanine, r-glutamylethylamide, on brain monoamines and striatal dopamine release in conscious rats. Neurochem Res. 1998;23:667–73.
67. Lardner AL. Neurobiological effects of the green tea constituent theanine and its potential role in the treatment of psychiatric and neurodegenerative disorders. Nutr Neurosci. 2014;17:145–55.
68. Heese T et al. Anxiolytic effects of L-theanine: a component of green tea-when combined with midazolam, in the male Sprague-Dawley rat. AANA J. 2009;77:445–9.
69. Kelly SP et al. L-theanine and caffeine in combination affect human cognition as evidenced by oscillatory alpha-band activity and attention task performance. J Nutr. 2008;138.
70. Wise LE et al. L-theanine attenuates abstinence signs in morphine-dependent rhesus monkeys and elicits anxiolytic-like activity in mice. Pharmacol Biochem Behav. 2012;103:245–52.
71. Banji D et al. Amelioration of behavioral aberrations and oxidative markers by green tea extract in valproate induced autism in animals. Brain Res. 2011;1410:141–51.
72. Kaur T et al. Effects of green tea extract on learning, memory, behavior and acetylcholinesterase activity in young and old male rats. Brain Cogn. 2008;67:25–30.
73. Bitu Pinto N et al. Neuroprotective properties of the standardized extract from Camellia sinensis (Green Tea) and its main bioactive components, Epicatechin and Epigallocatechin Gallate, in the 6-OHDA model of Parkinson's Disease. Evid Based Complement Alternat Med. 2015;2015.
74. Vignes M et al. Anxiolytic properties of green tea polyphenol (−)-epigallocatechin gallate (EGCG). Brain Res. 2006;1110:102–15.
75. Stringer M et al. Low dose EGCG treatment beginning in adolescence does not improve cognitive impairment in a Down syndrome mouse model. Pharmacol Biochem Behav. 2015:70–9.
76. Dodd FL et al. A double-blind, placebo-controlled study evaluating the effects of caffeine and L-theanine both alone and in combination on cerebral blood flow, cognition and mood. Psychopharmacology (Berl). 2015;232:2563–76.

77. Rogers PJ et al. Time for tea: mood, blood pressure and cognitive performance effects of caffeine and theanine administered alone and together. Psychopharmacology (Berl). 2008;195:569–77.
78. Camfield DA et al. Acute effects of tea constituents L-theanine, caffeine, and epigallocatechin gallate on cognitive function and mood: a systematic review and meta-analysis. Nutr Rev. 2014;72:507–22.
79. Ritsner MS et al. L-theanine relieves positive, activation, and anxiety symptoms in patients with schizophrenia and schizoaffective disorder: an 8-week, randomized, double-blind, placebo-controlled, 2-center study. J Clin Psychiatry. 2011;72(1):34–42.
80. White DJ et al. Anti-stress, behavioural and magnetoencephalography effects of an l-theanine-based nutrient drink: a randomised, double-blind, placebo-controlled, crossover trial. Nutrients. 2016;8.
81. Yoto A et al. Effects of L-theanine or caffeine intake on changes in blood pressure under physical and psychological stresses. J Physiol Anthropol. 2012;31:28.
82. Kimura K et al. l-Theanine reduces psychological and physiological stress responses. Biol Psychol. 2007;74(1):39–45.
83. Scholey A et al. Acute neurocognitive effects of epigallocatechin gallate (EGCG). Appetite. 2012;58:767–70.
84. Wightman EL et al. Epigallocatechin gallate, cerebral blood flow parameters, cognitive performance and mood in healthy humans: a double-blind, placebo-controlled, crossover investigation. Hum Psychopharmacol. 2012;27:177–86.
85. Borgwardt S et al. Neural effects of green tea extract on dorsolateral prefrontal cortex. Eur J Clin Nutr. 2012;66:1187–92.
86. Perry E, Howes MJR. Medicinal plants and dementia therapy: herbal hopes for brain aging? CNS Neurosci Ther. 2011;17:683–98.
87. Perry NSL et al. In-vitro inhibition of human erythrocyte acetylcholinesterase by Salvia lavandulaefolia essential oil and constituent terpenes. J Pharm Pharmacol. 2000;52:895–902.
88. Savelev S et al. Synergistic and antagonistic interactions of anticholinesterase terpenoids in Salvia lavandulaefolia essential oil. Pharmacol Biochem Behav. 2003;75:661–8.
89. Perry NSL et al. Salvia lavandulaefolia essential oil inhibits cholinesterase in vivo. Phytomedicine. 2002;9:48–51.
90. Savelev SU, Okello EJ, Perry EK. Butyryl- and acetyl-cholinesterase inhibitory activities in essential oils of Salvia species and their constituents. Phytother Res. 2004;18:315–24.
91. Perry NSL et al. Salvia for dementia therapy: review of pharmacological activity and pilot tolerability clinical trial. Pharmacol Biochem Behav. 2003;75:651–9.
92. Herrera-Ruiz M et al. Antidepressant and anxiolytic effects of hydroalcoholic extract from Salvia elegans. J Ethnopharmacol. 2006;107:53–8.
93. Mora S et al. The hydroalcoholic extract of Salvia elegans induces anxiolytic- and antidepressant-like effects in rats. J Ethnopharmacol. 2006;106:76–81.
94. Hosseinzadeh H, Danaee A, Ziaee T. Anti-anxiety effect of aqueous and ethanolic extracts of Salvia leriifolia Benth. leaves in mice using elevated plus maze. J Med Plants. 2008;7:25–36.
95. Rabbani M et al. Anxiolytic effects of Salvia reuterana Boiss. on the elevated plus-maze model of anxiety in mice. J Ethnopharmacol. 2005;101:100–3.
96. Liu AD et al. Anxiolytic effect of essential oils of Salvia miltiorrhiza in rats. Int J Clin Exp Med. 2015;8:12756–64.
97. Tildesley NTJ et al. Positive modulation of mood and cognitive performance following administration of acute doses of Salvia lavandulaefolia essential oil to healthy young volunteers. Physiol Behav. 2005;83:699–709.
98. Kennedy DO et al. Effects of cholinesterase inhibiting sage (Salvia officinalis) on mood, anxiety and performance on a psychological stressor battery. Neuropsychopharmacology. 2006;31:845–52.

99. Kennedy DO et al. Monoterpenoid extract of sage (Salvia lavandulaefolia) with cholinesterase inhibiting properties improves cognitive performance and mood in healthy adults. J Psychopharmacol. 2011;25:1088–100.
100. Eidi M, Eidi A, Bahar M. Effects of Salvia officinalis L. (sage) leaves on memory retention and its interaction with the cholinergic system in rats. Nutrition. 2006;22:321–6.
101. Tildesley NTJ et al. Salvia lavandulaefolia (Spanish sage) enhances memory in healthy young volunteers. Pharmacol Biochem Behav. 2003;75:669–74.
102. Scholey AB et al. An extract of Salvia (sage) with anticholinesterase properties improves memory and attention in healthy older volunteers. Psychopharmacology (Berl). 2008;198:127–39.
103. Akhondzadeh S et al. Salvia officinalis extract in the treatment of patients with mild to moderate Alzheimer's disease: a double blind, randomized and placebo-controlled trial. J Clin Pharm Ther. 2003;28:53–9.
104. El Omri A et al. Rosmarinus officinalis polyphenols activate cholinergic activities in PC12 cells through phosphorylation of ERK1/2. J Ethnopharmacol. 2010;131:451–8.
105. Orhan I et al. Inhibitory effect of Turkish Rosmarinus officinalis L. on acetylcholinesterase and butyrylcholinesterase enzymes. Food Chem. 2008;108:663–8.
106. Kovar KA et al. Blood levels of 1,8-cineole and locomotor activity of mice after inhalation and oral administration of rosemary oil. Planta Med. 1987;53:315–8.
107. Ozarowski M et al. Rosmarinus officinalis L. leaf extract improves memory impairment and affects acetylcholinesterase and butyrylcholinesterase activities in rat brain. Fitoterapia. 2013;91:261–71.
108. Heuberger E et al. Physiological and behavioral effects of 1,8-cineol and (±)-linalool: a comparison of inhalation and massage aromatherapy. Nat Prod Commun. 2008;3:1103–10.
109. Moss M et al. Aromas of rosemary and lavender essential oils differentially affect cognition and mood in healthy adults. Int J Neurosci. 2003;113:15–38.
110. Diego MA et al. Aromatherapy positively affects mood, EEG patterns of alertness and math computations. Int J Neurosci. 1998;96:217–24.
111. Tsang HW, Ho TY. A systematic review on the anxiolytic effects of aromatherapy on rodents under experimentally induced anxiety models. Rev Neurosci. 2010;21:141–52.
112. Ferlemi AV et al. Rosemary tea consumption results to anxiolytic- and anti-depressant-like behavior of adult male mice and inhibits all cerebral area and liver cholinesterase activity; phytochemical investigation and in silico studies. Chem Biol Interact. 2015;237:47–57.
113. Abdelhalim A et al. Antidepressant, anxiolytic and antinociceptive activities of constituents from rosmarinus officinalis. J Phar Pharm Sci. 2015;18:448–59.
114. McCaffrey R, Thomas DJ, Kinzelman AO. The effects of lavender and rosemary essential oils on test-taking anxiety among graduate nursing students. Holist Nurs Pract. 2009;23:88–93.
115. Rho KH et al. Effects of aromatherapy massage on anxiety and self-esteem in Korean elderly women: a pilot study. Int J Neurosci. 2006;116:1447–55.
116. Lee YL et al. A systematic review on the anxiolytic effects of aromatherapy in people with anxiety symptoms. J Altern Complement Med. 2011;17:101–8.
117. Burnett KM, Solterbeck LA, Strapp CM. Scent and mood state following an anxiety-provoking task. Psychol Rep. 2004;95:707–22.
118. Field T. Massage therapy research review. Complement Ther Clin Pract. 2014;20(4=):224–9.
119. Keeratitanont K et al. The efficacy of traditional Thai massage for the treatment of chronic pain: a systematic review. Complement Ther Clin Pract. 2015;21:26–32.
120. Yuan SLK, Matsutani LA, Marques AP. Effectiveness of different styles of massage therapy in fibromyalgia: a systematic review and meta-analysis. Man Ther. 2015;20:257–64.
121. Morin AK. Off-label use of atypical antipsychotic agents for treatment of insomnia. Mental Health Clinician (March 2014-Trends in Sedative-Hypnotic Therapy). 2014;4:65–72.
122. APA. Diagnostic and statistical manual of mental disorders. 5th ed. Arlington: American Psychiatric Publishing; 2013.

123. Beck AT. Cognitive therapy: basics and beyond. New York: Guilford Press; 1995.
124. Clark, D.A. and A.T. Beck, Cognitive therapy of anxiety disorders: science and practice. 2010, New York: Guilford Publications.
125. Barlow DH. Clinical handbook of psychological disorders: a step-by-step treatment manual. 4th ed. New York: The Guilford Press; 2008.
126. Bennett-Levy J et al. Oxford guide to behavioural experiments in cognitive therapy. Oxford, UK: Oxford University Press; 2004.

Nutritional-Based Nutraceuticals in the Treatment of Anxiety

5

David A. Camfield

5.1 Introduction

The term nutraceutical, which comes from a combination of the words 'nutrition' and 'pharmaceutical' [1], has been defined as 'a food (or part of a food) that provides medical or health benefits, including the prevention and/or treatment of a disease' [2]. However, in recent years, the use of the term has broadened beyond that of strictly food products, and in common practice is now typically used to refer to any over the counter nutritional substances and dietary supplements with medicinal effects. In the current chapter, these substances, rather than herbal extracts, will be the focus of discussion. Many nutraceuticals have been found to have acute and/or chronic neuropsychiatric effects, and varied mechanisms of action. These include antioxidant and anti-inflammatory effects, hypothalamic–pituitary–adrenal (HPA) axis regulation, together with more direct modulatory effects on neurotransmitter systems such as serotonin, dopamine and glutamate. Whilst clinical research into the efficacy of these substances in treating psychiatric disorders is still in its infancy, this emerging field of research has demonstrated great progress over the past 20 years. Promising lines of evidence suggest that the substances that are detailed in this chapter (B vitamins, magnesium, lysine, myo-inositol (MI) and N-acetylcysteine) have potential efficacy in reducing somatic, cognitive and affective anxiety symptoms across a range of disorders including panic disorder, obsessive-compulsive disorder (OCD), acute stress disorders and generalized anxiety disorder (GAD). Table 5.1 provides an overview of these nutritional medicines.

D.A. Camfield
School of Psychology, University of Wollongong, Wollongong, NSW, Australia

Centre for Human Psychopharmacology, Swinburne University of Technology, Hawthorn, VIC, Australia
e-mail: camfield@uow.edu.au

D. Camfield et al. (eds.), *Evidence-Based Herbal and Nutritional Treatments for Anxiety in Psychiatric Disorders*, DOI 10.1007/978-3-319-42307-4_5

Table 5.1 Nutritional substances with evidence of efficacy in the treatment of anxiety

Herbal medicine	Dosage	Mechanisms of action	Key evidence	Potential AEs	Potential clinical use	Clinical advice
MV/B vitamins	B9 > 800 µg B12 > 1 mg	HCy lowering, HPA axis regulation	MV consistently reduces stress in non-clinical samples	Check all listed constituents if taking a broad spectrum MV	Folic acid (B9) in depression Potential use of broad spectrum MV in acute stress disorders	Most effective for individuals with dietary deficiency, elderly or comorbid depression. Ensure adequate levels of B9 and B12
Magnesium	100–300 mg	Glutamate (NMDA inhibition)	Reduces anxious distress in depression. Also may be effective in GAD	Well tolerated with few side effects	Use in depression with anxious distress, as well as GAD, anxiety associated with premenstrual symptoms	More research required to differentiate magnesium effects from those of other substances (e.g. MVs). Magnesium oxide is not a very bioavailable form
L-lysine and L-arginine	2640–3000 mg/day	GABA, serotonin	Combined lysine/arginine reduces trait and state anxiety in non-clinical samples	Arginine may interact with some medications (e.g. blood pressure, Viagra)	Anxiety disorders, although further research required	Further research required, but may have potential efficacy

Myo-Inositol	12 g/day depression/ panic disorder 18 g/day OCD	Serotonin	Early studies suggest efficacy in panic disorder and OCD, when used as monotherapy	Gastrointestinal upset	Panic disorder (when used chronically), OCD (as monotherapy, without SSRIs)	Consumption of large quantity required. Soft gel capsules now available
N-Acetylcysteine	1200–3000 mg/day (although can take higher dose if need be)	Antioxidant (GSH enhancement) Glutamate modulation	OCD and related disorders, potential efficacy in GAD and social anxiety	Well tolerated with few side effects	OCD and grooming disorders, potentially GAD. Also effective in depression, bipolar disorder and substance use	Clinical effects are slow to develop, titration best if done gradually

MV: Multi-vitamin, GABA: Gamma-amino-butyric acid, HCy: Homocysteine, SSRI: Selective Serotonin Reuptake Inhibitor, GAD: Generalized Anxiety Disorder, GSH: Glutathione, OCD: Obsessive-Compulsive Disorder, HPA: Hyptohalamic-Pituitary-Adrenal Axis, NMDA: N-methyl-D-aspartate, AE: Adverse Event

5.2 B Vitamins

5.2.1 Overview

B vitamins can be obtained from dietary sources in addition to supplement form. The majority of previous research has focussed on the vitamins pyridoxine (B6), folic acid (B9) and cobalamin/cyanocobalamin (B12). These have been found to be rapidly absorbed when taken orally, with peak plasma levels observed within the first 3 h post-dose [3–5], indicating that acute as well as chronic effects may be expected.

5.2.2 Mechanisms of Action (Constituents)

Vitamins B6, B9 and B12 perform a number of important functions in the human brain, including acting as cofactors in neurotransmitter synthesis, glucocorticoid (stress hormone) production and the conversion of homocysteine (HCy) back to methionine [6–9]. S-adenosylmethionine (SAMe) is the most important methyl donor in the human body, with HCy being a by-product of its methylation (refer to Chap. 6 for further details on mood effects associated with SAMe). Folic acid (B9) and B12 are co-factors required to recycle HCy back to methionine, and without adequate levels of these vitamins, methylation processes are impaired [8] and HCy accumulates in the body. HCy accumulation is associated with a range of adverse physiological effects including increased oxidative stress, neuronal excitotoxicity, DNA strand breakage, production of amyloid precursor protein (APP; implicated in the development of Alzheimer's disease) and mitochondrial membrane damage [10–12]. Further, genetic differences in the methylenetetrahydrofolate reductase (MTHFR) gene result in some individuals being more susceptible to HCy accumulation than others. In particular, the 677 TT polymorphism of the MTHFR gene, which relates to reduced enzymatic metabolism of HCy, has been found to be associated with an increased risk of depression. Research regarding the mechanism of action of the other B vitamins is ongoing; for example, a recent preclinical study found B1 to increase brain-derived neurotrophic factor (BDNF) levels in an animal model of stress [13], and a recent review by Kennedy [14] suggests that eight of the B vitamins have closely inter-related functions, and are important for optimal neurological function.

5.2.3 Evidence of Efficacy

The majority of research regarding the psychopharmacology of B vitamins (and multi-vitamins (MVs) more generally) has been conducted in non-clinical samples, and whilst these findings may not be able to directly prove efficacy for individuals with clinically significant anxiety, it is nevertheless informative that these studies have consistently demonstrated reductions in stress together with improved mood.

5.2.3.1 Stress Reduction and Mood Improvements (Non-Clinical)

The stress-reducing effects of B vitamins may be attributable to modulation of HCy accumulation, as well as glucocorticoid production, and possible modulatory effects on the HPA axis. Preliminary evidence also suggests that MV supplementation containing B vitamins may modulate cortisol levels, as indicated by elevation of the cortisol awakening response [15]. In a large randomised-controlled trial (RCT) by Schlebusch et al. [16], 300 adults reporting high levels of stress were administered a vitamin B complex (Berocca Calmag; including 8.25 mg B6, and 10 μg B12) for 30 days, with reduced psychological distress (as measured by the Berocca® Stress Index, Hamilton Anxiety Rating Scale and Psychological General Well-Being Scale) reported in comparison to placebo. Another study by Carroll et al. (2000) found reductions in stress levels (measured by the perceived stress scale; PSS), in psychological distress (according to the General Health Questionnaire; GHQ-28) and in anxiety symptoms (measured by the Hospital Anxiety and Depression Scale; HADS). The reduction in these symptoms occurred following 4 weeks of supplementation with a MV containing B vitamins (Berocca® including 10 mg B6, 400 μg B9 and 10 μg B12) in 80 healthy males. Similarly, Stough et al. [17] also reported that 3-month supplementation with a high-dose vitamin B complex (including 20.63 mg B6, 150 μg B9 and 30 μg B12) in 60 participants reporting chronic work-related stress was associated with lowered ratings of personal strain as measured by the Occupational Stress Inventory.

A number of studies have demonstrated similar findings regarding stress, fatigue and other mood measures [18–24]. A meta-analysis by Long and Benton [25] reported that chronic MV supplementation in non-clinical samples was associated with reduced levels of perceived stress (Standardized Mean Difference; SMD = 0.35), anxiety (SMD = 0.32), fatigue (SMD = 0.27), confusion (SMD = 0.23) and mild psychiatric symptoms (SMD = 0.30). No evidence for a reduction in depressive symptoms was found in the non-clinical samples, although the supplements containing higher doses of B vitamins were found to be more effective in improving mood states.

5.2.3.2 Depression

In regards to clinically significant depression, a number of large epidemiological studies have linked deficiencies in B9 and B12, together with elevated HCy levels with a higher incidence of depressive disorders [26–30]. Similarly, an animal study by Botez et al. [31] found an association between folate deficiency and reduced brain serotonin synthesis. A few intervention studies have also been published in relation to folate in depressed samples. An early placebo-controlled trial by Godfrey et al. [32] in 43 patients with folate deficiency (<200 μg/l red-cell folate) and a DSM III diagnosis of major depression or schizophrenia reported that 15 mg/day of folic acid (in addition to standard psychotropic treatments) for 6 months was associated with improved clinical and social outcomes.

In a randomized study by Passeri et al. [33], 50 mg/day of 5′-Methyltetrahydrofolic acid (5′-MTHF) for 8 weeks was found to be equally effective as 100 mg/day trazodone in reducing depressive symptoms in 96 elderly participants with dementia and depression, as measured using the Hamilton Depression Rating Scale (HDRS). In an augmentation study with 0.5 mg folic acid/day in addition to fluoxetine (20 mg/

day) in 127 patients with a DSM III-R diagnosis of major depression, Coppen and Bailey [34] reported a greater proportion of female treatment responders (>50 % reduction in HDRS score) in the folic acid group in comparison to placebo augmentation (93.3 % versus 61.1 %, respectively). Plasma HCy levels were also significantly reduced in women (20.6 %). Interestingly, no significant clinical effects or HCy effects were found in men, with the authors suggesting that the effective dose may have been insufficient to observe treatment effects in males. In a smaller open-label study by Alpert et al. [35], 15–30 mg/day of folinic acid (Leucovorin) was added to existing selective serotonin reuptake inhibitor (SSRI) treatment over an 8-week period in 22 adults with a DSM-IV diagnosis of major depressive disorder (MDD). Significant reductions in the HDRS scores were observed for treatment completers ($n = 17$), although only 27 % of the intention-to-treat sample achieved a treatment response (<50 % reduction in HDRS scores). In a meta-analysis of the findings from these three folate intervention studies, Taylor et al. [36] found that adding folate to existing treatments (e.g. SSRIs) resulted in an average reduction of an extra 2.65 points on the HDRS. In a subsequent narrative review of folic acid and B12 in the treatment of depression, Coppen et al. [37] recommended that 800 μg/day of folic acid (B9) and 1 mg/day of vitamin B12 be utilized in future intervention studies.

5.2.3.3 Anxiety

In relation to the effects of B vitamin supplementation in addressing clinically significant anxiety symptoms, there is currently a paucity of published findings. However, an intriguing study by Rucklidge and colleagues [38, 39] provided evidence of MV supplementation with B vitamins providing beneficial effects in the aftermath of a 6.3 earthquake in Christchurch New Zealand, 2011. Ninety-one adults reporting heightened anxiety or stress 2 to 3 months following the earthquake were randomized to 28 days of Berocca™ (including 10 mg B6, 400 μg B9 and 10 μg B12) or varying doses of a MV (CNE) containing B vitamins (maximum doses of 19.2 mg B6, 768 μg B9 and 480 μg B12). However, it should be noted that a large range of other nutraceutical substances were also included in the CNE supplements. All groups were found to have significant reductions in symptoms of psychological distress, as measured by the Depression and Anxiety Scale (DASS), Impact of Event Scale (IES-R) and Perceived Stress Scale (PSS), with greater improvements in mood, anxiety and energy observed in the high-dose CME group when compared to Berocca™. Whilst these findings are encouraging, they need be interpreted conservatively in consideration of the lack of a placebo comparator group. It is also noteworthy that the broad range MV demonstrated greater efficacy than the Berooca™ high-dose vitamin B complex, suggesting that other substances may have been responsible for the effect (see section on magnesium below). In a 1-year follow-up study, Rucklidge et al. [39] reported that participants who were involved in the study and received Berocca™ or CME treatment ($n = 64$) had better long-term outcomes compared with controls who had not received the treatment ($n = 21$).

In summary, further research is required in regards to the efficacy of supplementation with MV and B vitamins in the amelioration of clinical depression, anxiety and stress symptoms. B vitamins, in particular folate (B9) and B12, appear to have efficacy in reducing stress and improving mood in non-clinical adult samples. There is evidence to suggest that folate (B9) may be effective as an adjunct treatment for participants with depression, particularly in cases of folate deficiency. In regards to the effects of MV and B vitamin supplementation in anxiety, the studies by Rucklidge et al. [38, 39] provide intriguing preliminary data regarding the potential efficacy of these substances in ameliorating the effects of trauma and stressor-related anxiety and stress. Further research in clinical samples is warranted, together with a more detailed analysis of the relative contribution of each substance to reductions in clinical symptoms. MTHFR genotyping would also be informative, regarding whether supplementation with B vitamins is more effective for individuals with the 677 TT polymorphism.

5.3 Magnesium

5.3.1 Overview

Magnesium is an essential element that is used extensively throughout the body, being required as a cofactor in over 300 enzymatic reactions, as well as for the production of ATP and nucleic acids [40]. Magnesium is readily obtained through dietary sources, although deficiency may occur with poor diet, partly due to the reduced amounts now contained in modern diets which consist of largely refined and processed foods [41, 42]. Magnesium can be taken as a supplement in various forms, the most readily available form in Western countries being magnesium oxide (although more bioavailable ligands are also available, see clinical considerations at the end of the chapter).

5.3.2 Mechanisms of Action

Magnesium is an inhibitor of *N*-methyl-D-aspartate (NMDA) glutamate receptors, where activation of the NMDA receptor ion channel is blocked by magnesium in a voltage-dependent manner [43]. Antidepressant as well as anxiolytic effects have been attributed to this glutamatergic mechanism, as investigated in animal models such as the forced swim and the elevated plus-maze (EPM) test [44, 45]. Additional mechanisms of action have also been postulated, including modulatory effects on the HPA axis [46], as well as inhibition of the GSK-3 enzyme [47]. Clinical data suggest that there are lower plasma magnesium levels in depressed [48] and anxious patients [49], and lower cerebrospinal fluid (CSF) levels of magnesium in those who are suicidal [50]. There is also limited evidence to suggest that magnesium may be of assistance in reducing premenstrual symptoms (PMS) and associated distress, with supplemental magnesium intake likely to help restore magnesium deficiency as a result of blood loss, as well as having a sedative effect on neuromuscular excitability and aiding in the restoration of electrolyte imbalances within cell membranes [51].

5.3.3 Evidence of Efficacy

A series of four case studies were presented by Eby and Eby [46] regarding the use of magnesium in the treatment of depression. Rapid recovery in less than 7 days was documented in all cases, using doses of 125–300 mg magnesium (as glycinate or taurinate) with each meal and at bedtime. Of particular interest was that comorbid symptoms of anxiety, agitation and irritability were also found to be reduced following magnesium supplementation. De Souza et al. [52] conducted a randomized placebo-controlled cross-over study comparing the effects of 200 mg magnesium (magnesium oxide) with 50 mg vitamin B6 in 44 women with mild premenstrual symptoms. Participants received each treatment, as well as their combination, for one menstrual cycle per treatment. The combined magnesium and B6 treatment was associated with a significant reduction in anxiety-related premenstrual symptoms (i.e. nervous tension, mood swings, irritability or anxiety) as measured by the Menstrual Health Questionnaire (MHQ). The authors attributed these findings to a synergistic effect of B6 and magnesium, whereby B6 facilitated magnesium absorption. In regards to the non-significant findings of magnesium when administered by itself, the authors suggested that a longer period of supplementation may have been required for increased magnesium absorption. However, it is noteworthy that in a previous study in 38 women from the same group [53], 2-month supplementation with 200 mg magnesium was not found to be associated with any reductions in anxiety-related premenstrual symptoms, only in regards to hydration symptoms.

In a large double-blind, RCT of 264 patients with a DSM III-R diagnosis of GAD with mild-to-moderate severity, Hanus et al. [54] administered a combination of hawthorn (*Crateagus oxyacantha*, 75 mg), California poppy (*Eschscholtzia californica*, 20 mg) and magnesium (heavy magnesium oxide, 124.35 mg) for 90 days. Significant reductions in total and somatic Hamilton Anxiety Scale scores, as well as subjective patient-rated anxiety, were observed at study endpoint. However, it is difficult to ascertain the relative contribution of magnesium in comparison to the herbal constituents in this study.

It is noteworthy that magnesium is routinely included in most MV preparations, including those discussed in the previous section on B vitamins. For example, the Berocca™ formulation as used in the studies by Rucklidge [38, 39] and Schlebusch [16] contains 100 mg magnesium. Similarly, the CME formulation used in the study by Rucklidge et al. [38] contained a maximum dose of 320 mg magnesium, whereas the B vitamin complex administered in the study by Stough et al. [17] contained 140 mg of magnesium phosphate. Clearly, further research is required in order to better differentiate the psychopharmacological effects of magnesium from those associated with B vitamins and other nutrients.

5.4 Lysine and Arginine

5.4.1 Overview

L-lysine and L-arginine are amino acids which have been found to be beneficial in animal models of stress and anxiety, due to their modulatory effects on neurotransmitter systems including serotonin and GABA [55]. Lysine and arginine may be obtained from dietary sources such as dairy products and meats. Whilst arginine can be synthesized in the human body, it is not made in sufficient quantities to meet metabolic requirements during periods of stress [56].

5.4.2 Mechanisms of Action

Lysine has been found to act as a partial antagonist at serotonin 5-HT_4 receptors [57], and also interacts with central benzodiazepine receptors [58]. Arginine is a precursor for the production of nitric oxide (NO), and has been found to reverse the effects of restraint stress exposure in rodents [59]. Further, animal research suggests that combined lysine and arginine administration may aid in lowering cortisol levels and block anxiogenic responses to stressors [60].

5.4.3 Evidence of Efficacy

Jezova et al. [61] administered 3 g/day L-lysine and 3 g/day L-arginine (in gelatin capsules) versus placebo over a 10-day period to 29 healthy participants who reported high levels of trait anxiety according to the State-Trait Anxiety Inventory (STAI-T). Following the supplementation period, the participants' were exposed to a modified version of the Social Stress Test involving a 15 min speech. Higher neuroendocrine activation, as measured by cortisol, adrenaline, noradrenaline and adreno-corticotropic hormone (ACTH), was observed in the participants treated with the amino acid combination. The authors explained this finding as a normalization of a previously blunted stress response in the highly anxious participants.

In a large double-blind RCT of 108 healthy Japanese adults, Smriga et al. [62] administered 2.64 g/day L-lysine and 2.64 g/day L-arginine over a 7-day period. In response to a cognitive stress battery, both trait anxiety (STAI-T) and state anxiety (STAI-S) were significantly reduced following the amino acid treatment. Salivary cortisol and chromogranin-A levels were also found to be reduced in the male participants. These results corroborated the findings of a previous study by this group, which found that 3-month consumption of L-lysine fortified wheat similarly resulted in a reduction in trait anxiety (STAI-T) in males, and also reduced cortisol responses to a blood drawing (a culturally appropriate stressor) amongst low socioeconomic Syrian households [63]. However, it is important to note that this study involved individuals with a dietary deficiency in amino acids including lysine and arginine. Whilst this preliminary research is intriguing, further research is required in order to better determine if lysine and/or arginine supplementation are beneficial in the treatment of anxiety in clinical samples.

5.5 Myo-Inositol (MI)

5.5.1 Overview

Myo-Inositol (MI) is an endogenous isomer of glucose that is readily available in a powdered form and can be dissolved in water to result in a sweet-tasting drink. MI can be obtained in the diet from items such as fruits, beans, grains and nuts, but the quantities are small (typically 225–1500 mg/day per 1800 kcal [64].

5.5.2 Mechanisms of Action (Constituents)

Exogenous MI has been found to elevate levels of MI in both cerebrospinal fluid (CSF) and the brain [65], where it is stored predominantly in astrocytes [66]. Early studies in humans suggested that an oral MI dose of 12 g is sufficient to cross the blood–brain barrier, and raises the MI level in CSF by 70 % [67]. In regards to antidepressant and anxiolytic mechanisms of action, MI is an important precursor in the phosphoinositide (PI) secondary messenger system, which is involved in a number of neurotransmitter systems in the human brain including acetylcholine, noradrenaline and most notably serotonin. It has been theorized that MI modulates serotonergic function via a number of effects, including 5-HT receptor sensitization [68] and 5-HT transporter reuptake inhibition [69, 70]. The 5-HT_2 receptor class has also been specifically implicated in animal studies [71, 72]. The range of disorders in which MI efficacy has been reported and the time lag for its antidepressant effects (>4 weeks) are similar to those reported for SSRIs [73]. The interested reader is referred to Harvey et al. [72] and Camfield et al. [74] for a more detailed discussion of its mechanisms of action. Side effects associated with MI administration are generally mild [75]; however, mild gastrointestinal side effects in the first 2 weeks of treatment have been reported in some patients, including diarrhoea, flatulence, bloating and nausea [76].

5.5.2.1 Evidence of Efficacy

MI has been found to have acute effects on mood within 6 h post-dose [77], and the antidepressant effects of MI in clinical samples, including MDD and premenstrual dysphoric disorder (PMDD), have been well supported across a number of studies [78]. In regards to the efficacy of MI as an anxiolytic, there has been some preliminary research conducted in regards to panic disorder, post-traumatic stress disorder (PTSD) and obsessive-compulsive disorder (OCD).

5.5.2.2 Panic Disorder

Benefits associated with chronic MI consumption have been reported for panic disorder in two studies. In the first study, Benjamin et al. [79] administered 12 g/day MI (6 g/day BID, dissolved in juice) versus placebo to 21 individuals with a DSM III-R diagnosis of panic disorder (16 with agoraphobia), in a 4-week double-blind cross-over trial. The frequency and severity of panic attacks as well as agoraphobic symptoms declined significantly more following MI treatment than placebo. In a subsequent double-blind cross-over comparator study, 20 patients with a DSM-IV diagnosis of panic disorder (with or without agoraphobia) were administered a maximum dose of 18 g/day of MI versus 150 mg/day fluvoxamine for 4 weeks. Improvements on Hamilton Rating Scale for Anxiety, agoraphobia scores and Clinical Global Impression (CGI) of change were similar for both treatments. Further, MI was found to reduce the number of panic attacks (4.0/week) to a greater extent than fluvoxamine (2.4/week), and side effects of nausea and tiredness were also more common with fluvoxamine. In regards to acute effects of MI in ameliorating the effects of panic symptoms, Benjamin et al. [80] reported no effect when a single 20 g dose of MI or placebo was administered to seven patients who met DSM-IV criteria for panic disorder. Panic symptoms were pharmaceutically induced using a known panicogen, meta-chlorophenylpiperazine (intravenous m-CPP), with DSM-IV panic symptom scores together with cortisol and pupil sizes not found to be differentially effected by MI. However, it should be noted that this study was underpowered, and the authors note that the study's findings do not preclude the possibility that chronic MI administration may ameliorate symptoms in the m-CPP challenge test.

5.5.2.3 Post-traumatic Stress Disorder (PTSD)

In regards to PTSD, there is currently no evidence to support the use of MI as monotherapy in the treatment of this complex disorder. Kaplan et al. [81] administered 12 g/day MI or placebo to 13 patients who met DSM-III-R criteria for PTSD over a 4-week period in a randomized cross-over trial. No significant improvements were found for MI, according to the Impact of Event Scale (IES), including both intrusion and avoidance trauma symptoms.

5.5.2.4 Obsessive-Compulsive Disorder (OCD)

A series of initial studies were conducted to investigate MI as a possible treatment for OCD. Fux et al. [82] administered 18 g/day MI to 13 OCD patients (DSM-IV diagnosis) over a period of 6 weeks in a double-blind, randomized, placebo-controlled, cross-over design, using glucose as a placebo. Scores on the Yale-Brown Obsessive Compulsive Scale (Y-BOCS) were found to be significantly reduced for the MI group compared to placebo at study endpoint. However, in a follow-up augmentation study by the same group in 10 DSM-IV diagnosed OCD patients, MI was found to be ineffective in reducing obsessive-compulsive symptoms when 18 g/day MI was added to an existing SSRI regimen (fluoxetine, fluvoxamine or clomipramine) for 6 weeks [83]. The authors interpreted this lack of significant benefit as indicating that SSRIs and MI have overlapping modes of action (i.e. serotonergic enhancements). Seedat et al. [84] also reported no advantage for MI versus placebo in an open-label augmentation study where 18 g/day MI was administered to treatment-refractory OCD patients in conjunction with high-dose SSRI treatment (fluoxetine, sertraline, clomipramine or citalopram). Whilst it was noteworthy that a small decrease in Y-BOCS scores was observed in the group as a whole, the majority of patients (7/10) did not improve, as measured by the Clinical Global Impression (CGI) scale.

A more recent open-label study by Carey et al. [76] in 14 treatment-free DSM-IV diagnosed OCD patients reported a significant reduction in Y-BOCS scores and Clinical Global Impression of change (CGI) when MI was administered at 18 g/day for 12 weeks. Changes in brain perfusion, as measured by single photon emission computed tomography (SPECT), were also observed across a number of regions at study endpoint. In relation to symptom reduction in the related disorders of trichotillomania (compulsive hair pulling; TTM) and excoriation (compulsive skin picking), Seedat et al. [85] reported clinical responses to MI in three patients. All three cases showed substantial improvement on 18 g/day MI, as measured on the CGI.

It is noteworthy that the use of 18 g/day of MI has not been well justified in the literature. Early studies by Levine [67, 86] suggested that 12 g/day of MI may be an effective dose for the treatment of depression; therefore, it is unclear as to why 18 g/day was decided for subsequent studies of MI in the treatment of OCD. Presumably, the 18 mg dose was arbitrarily determined by the fact that higher doses of SSRIs are typically required for treatment response in OCD compared to depression. However, to date no systematic dose-escalation study has been conducted in order to determine appropriate dose ranges for this disorder. For this reason, it is possible that a higher dose of MI is required for clinically significant effects in OCD patients with more severe presentations.

Despite the initial enthusiasm for MI as a treatment for OCD, there has been no further research examining its efficacy. The existing clinical evidence suggests that MI at a dose of 18 g/day may potentially be effective as monotherapy for OCD, whilst there is currently no evidence to suggest that it adds additional benefit above and beyond ongoing SSRI treatment. Further research is needed, due to the fact that these early studies examined only a single dose (18 g) and only involved patients with moderately severe symptoms.

5.6 N-Acetylcysteine (NAC)

5.6.1 Overview

NAC is a derivative of the amino acid L-cysteine, and is a good oral source of cysteine due to it being more water soluble, less reactive, less toxic and less susceptible to oxidation in comparison to cysteine itself [87]. NAC is not found through regular dietary sources, so is taken as a dietary supplement.

5.6.2 Mechanism of Action

NAC is rapidly absorbed, with time to peak plasma levels (t_{max}) being 1.4 ± 0.7 h following oral administration, and an elimination half-life ($t_{1/2}$) of 2.5 ± 0.6 h [88]. The bioavailability of NAC increases according to the dose, with the peak serum level being on average 16 μmol/l after 600 mg and 35 μmol/l after 1200 mg [89]. NAC is absorbed by the stomach and intestines, where a large proportion is converted to cysteine in the liver [90]. There has been some inconsistency in the literature regarding the ability of NAC (as well as cysteine) to cross the blood–brain barrier [91]; however, a recent human study reported biologically relevant increases in CSF NAC and cysteine concentrations within 90 min of oral dosing [92].

The two primary mechanisms of action that have been investigated in relation to the neuropsychiatric effects of NAC involve the inhibition of synaptic glutamate release via actions at the cystine-glutamate antiporter on glial cells [93], and increased production of the endogenous antioxidant glutathione (GSH), which results in a reduction in brain oxidative stress and inflammation [94, 95]. There is also evidence to suggest that NAC may work well as an adjunct to antidepressant therapy, with preclinical data suggesting that NAC may lower their effective dose [96]. NAC is generally well tolerated, with a low incidence of adverse events in doses up to 8000 mg/day [97]; in a review of over 46 placebo-controlled trials, no significant adverse effects were reported [90].

5.6.3 Evidence of Efficacy

Over the past decade, the treatment effects of NAC have been studied in a wide range of psychiatric disorders, perhaps more so than any other nutraceutical substance in psychiatry—with evidence of efficacy found for bipolar disorder, substance abuse, depression, schizophrenia and obsessive-compulsive spectrum disorders, among others [98, 99].

5.6.3.1 Generalized Anxiety Disorder and Social Phobia

In relation to the treatment of anxiety disorders, RCTs of NAC are yet to be conducted. However, preliminary evidence of potential efficacy was provided in a single case study by Strawn and Saldaña [100] involving a 17-year-old male with GAD and social phobia. The patient was experiencing some relief from high-dose (150 mg/day) sertraline, yet still experienced significant anxiety and functional impairment, with a Clinical Global Impression Scale (CGI-S) score of 5. NAC 1200 mg/day was initiated, in addition to sertraline, for 4 weeks, before being titrated up to 2400 mg/day for another 4 weeks (8 weeks in total). Clinical response was rapid, with reductions in somatic and psychological anxiety symptoms within 1 week, and by the end of 8 weeks adjunctive NAC, his CGI-S had decreased to 2, and improvements were noted in symptoms of insomnia, restlessness, inner tension and somatic anxiety symptoms. He was subsequently able to recommence social activities with friends and apply for part-time employment.

5.6.3.2 Obsessive-Compulsive and Related Disorder

OCD is a disorder which has been associated with increased levels of oxidative stress, lipid peroxidation and elevated levels of pro-inflammatory cytokines [101–103]. For this reason, the powerful antioxidant effects of NAC may be of benefit in this disorder [94, 104]. In addition, NAC's inhibitory effects on synaptic glutamate release may also be of benefit, due to abnormally elevated levels of glutamate transmission observed in OCD, as reflected by hyperactivation within cortico-striatal-thalamo-cortical (CSTC) neurocircuits [93].

In a case report of a 58-year-old women with treatment-resistant OCD, Lafleur et al. [105] reported a large reduction in Y-BOCS symptom severity (from a baseline score of 32 to an endpoint score of 9) with 3000 mg/day NAC over a 12-week period. Although, in a subsequent case series by Van Ameringen et al. [106], only one patient in six reported a response with 4 weeks of 3000 mg/day NAC. In a randomized controlled trial in 48 OCD patients by Afshar et al. [107], 12-week NAC at a dose of 2400 mg/day was found to be associated with a significant Y-BOCS reduction from 8 weeks onwards, and a full clinical response in 10 out of 19 patients. In contrast, no significant benefit of NAC over placebo was found in a recent trial by Sarris et al. [108], where 44 patients with DSM-5 diagnosed OCD were administered NAC (3000 mg/day) or placebo over 16 weeks. However, further analysis revealed age to be a moderating factor, with a significant reduction in Y-BOCS scores in patients under 34 years, as well as a negative relationship between illness duration and treatment efficacy—which was indicative of reduced effects in more chronic sufferers [109]. A larger 16-week RCT using NAC in the treatment of OCD by Sarris and colleagues at the University of Melbourne has recently been funded (NHMRC APP1104460).

Evidence of efficacy for NAC in the treatment of related compulsive grooming disorders has also been reported in the literature, these include compulsive nail-biting [110, 111], compulsive hair-pulling [Trichotillomania; 112, 113, 114] and compulsive skin-picking [115]. In summary, preliminary evidence is supportive of NAC in the treatment of OCD; although, a number of issues still require resolution including whether it is effective in more severe presentations, and whether it works best as monotherapy or in addition to existing SSRI treatments [116].

5.7 Clinical Considerations

Further research in clinical samples is currently required in regards to the B vitamins, magnesium, arginine and lysine. Whilst promising preliminary research in non-clinical samples has provided evidence to suggest they may be effective in reducing stress and anxiety in otherwise healthy individuals, it remains to be established as to whether they are potent enough for addressing anxiety symptoms which are associated with clinically significant distress. However, it could also be argued that in clinical disorders where the pathological processes such as oxidative stress and HPA axis dysregulation are heightened, there may be an increased need for these substances. In either case, there is a strong argument for supplementation in cases of dietary insufficiency, such as in low socio-economic regions or elderly individuals. In regard to magnesium, the oxide form is most commonly available in Western countries [46]. However, the bioavailability for magnesium oxide in the human body has been found to be low in comparison to other highly biologically available forms of magnesium, including magnesium-chloride, −sulphate, −citrate, −lactate, −malate, −glycinate and -taurinate [117–119]. In the case of arginine, caution should be exercised in certain cases. Whilst arginine has generally been found to provide beneficial effects in relation to cardiovascular health [120], it can lower blood pressure and for this reason may be problematic when taken in conjunction with some blood pressure and heart medications, as well as Viagra. Arginine may also lower blood sugar levels, so for this reason should be used with caution in patients with type 2 diabetes who take insulin [121].

In the case of MI, mild gastrointestinal effects, including diarrhoea, flatulence, bloating and nausea, are commonly reported in the first 2 weeks of treatment [75] [76], which may be a deterrence to some individuals. From a practical perspective, taking 18 g of powder per day mixed into drinks over an extended period of time may also be inconvenient, and requires purchasing MI in large quantities (e.g. >1 kg) in order to maintain a stable supply. However, MI has also become available more recently in a soft gel capsule form, with 600 mg being roughly the same as 2 g of powder, with equivalent efficacy reported in terms of mood effects [122]. Also, due to MIs serotonergic mechanism of action, caution also needs to be exercised if using in conjunction with pharmaceutical antidepressants, St. John's wort or other serotoninergic enhancers. Whilst to the best of our knowledge no cases of serotonin syndrome have been reported in relation to MI use, if hypomanic symptoms develop then it would be wise to discontinue its use.

In regards to NAC, it is remarkably well tolerated at doses considerably higher than the 3 g/day upper limit reported in most clinical studies. However, it is not necessarily the case that higher doses provide a better clinical effect for any given individual. It is recommended that treatment commence with an initial low dose, either 600 mg or 1200 mg per day, and that the dose be slowly increased in 2-week intervals if need be. It is also important that expectations be managed appropriately in regards to potential antidepressant, anxiolytic or anti-obsessional effects. As a general rule, the majority of studies that have demonstrated efficacy for NAC in psychiatric disorders have involved chronic administration over a duration of 4 months or more [98, 99]; consequently, research to date suggests that the clinical effects of NAC are slow to develop. NAC can perhaps best be understood as a long-term maintenance treatment, aimed at improving brain health in the context of detrimental processes such as inflammation, oxidative stress and glutamate dysregulation. In regards to all substances reviewed in this chapter, it is important to obtain high-quality supplements that have been produced according to good manufacturing practice standards.

Finally, there are no known contra-indications for the use of these nutraceutical substances in conjunction with psychotherapeutic interventions such as cognitive–behavioural therapy for anxiety disorders, exposure and response prevention for OCD, or exposure-based treatments for PTSD. It could be argued that these substances, due to having a more gradual onset of action, represent a better match for conducting psychotherapeutic work. However, in the case of patients with severe presentations that are associated with high risk, such as suicidal ideation, then pharmaceutical alternatives with a more rapid onset are advised.

In summary, promising preliminary research suggests that the nutraceutical treatments of MI and NAC may have efficacy in the treatment of anxiety disorders, as well as obsessive compulsive and related disorders—although further research is required regarding dosage, duration and whether these substances are best used as monotherapy or adjunctive treatments. Whilst B vitamins have been found to be efficacious in reducing stress and anxiety in non-clinical samples, further research is required in order to investigate their efficacy in clinical disorders other than depression. Similarly, further research is also required in regards to the use of magnesium and the amino acids L-lysine and L-arginine in the treatment of anxiety associated with clinical disorders.

References

1. Kalra EK. Nutraceutical – definition and introduction. AAPS PharmSci. 2003;5(3).
2. Brower V. Nutraceuticals: poised for a healthy slice of the healthcare market? Nat Biotechnol. 1998;16(8):728–30.
3. Bor MV et al. Plasma vitamin B6 vitamers before and after oral vitamin B6 treatment: a randomized placebo-controlled study. Clin Chem. 2003;49(1):155–61.
4. Dainty JR et al. Quantification of the bioavailability of riboflavin from foods by use of stable-isotope labels and kinetic modeling. Am J Clin Nutr. 2007;85(6):1557–64.
5. Mönch S et al. Quantitation of folates and their catabolites in blood plasma, erythrocytes, and urine by stable isotope dilution assays. Anal Biochem. 2010;398(2):150–60.
6. Bottiglieri T. Homocysteine and folate metabolism in depression. Prog Neuropsychopharmacol Biol Psychiatry. 2005;29(7):1103–12.
7. Mattson MP, Shea TB. Folate and homocysteine metabolism in neural plasticity and neurodegenerative disorders. Trends Neurosci. 2003;26(3):137–46.
8. Miller AL. The methionine-homocysteine cycle and its effects on cognitive diseases. Altern Med Rev. 2003;8(1):7–19.
9. Head KA, Kelly GS. Nutrients and botanicals for treatment of stress: adrenal fatigue, neurotransmitter imbalance, anxiety, and restless sleep. Altern Med Rev. 2009;14(2):114–40.
10. Rogaev EI et al. The upstream promoter of the Î^2-amyloid precursor protein gene (APP) shows differential patterns of methylation in human brain. Genomics. 1994;22(2):340–7.
11. West RL, Lee JM, Maroun LE. Hypomethylation of the amyloid precursor protein gene in the brain of an alzheimer's disease patient. J Mol Neurosci. 1995;6(2):141–6.
12. Kruman II et al. Homocysteine elicits a DNA damage response in neurons that promotes apoptosis and hypersensitivity to excitotoxicity. J Neurosci. 2000;20(18):6920–6.

13. Dief AE, Samy DM, Dowedar FI. Impact of exercise and vitamin B1 intake on hippocampal brain-derived neurotrophic factor and spatial memory performance in a rat model of stress. J Nutr Sci Vitaminol. 2015;61(1):1–7.
14. Kennedy DO. B vitamins and the brain: Mechanisms, dose and efficacy—A review. Nutrients. 2016;8(2).
15. Camfield DA et al. The effects of multivitamin supplementation on diurnal cortisol secretion and perceived stress. Nutrients. 2013;5(11):4429–50.
16. Schlebusch L et al. A double-blind, placebo-controlled, double-centre study of the effects of an oral multivitamin-mineral combination on stress. S Afr Med J. 2000;90(12):1216–23.
17. Carroll D et al. The effects of an oral multivitamin combination with calcium, magnesium, and zinc on psychological well-being in healthy young male volunteers: A double-blind placebo-controlled trial. Psychopharmacology, 2000;150(2):220–225.
18. Stough C et al. The effect of 90 day administration of a high dose vitamin B-complex on work stress. Hum Psychopharmacol. 2011;26(7):470–6.
19. Harris E et al. Effects of a multivitamin, mineral and herbal supplement on cognition and blood biomarkers in older men: a randomised, placebo-controlled trial. Hum Psychopharmacol. 2012;27:370–7.
20. Macpherson H et al. Acute mood but not cognitive improvements following administration of a single multivitamin and mineral supplement in healthy women aged 50 and above: a randomised controlled trial. Age. 2015;37(3).
21. White DJ et al. Effects of four-week supplementation with a multi-vitamin/mineral preparation on mood and blood biomarkers in young adults: a randomised, double-blind, placebo-controlled trial. Nutrients. 2015;7(11):9005–17.
22. Haskell CF et al. Effects of a multi-vitamin/mineral supplement on cognitive function and fatigue during extended multi-tasking. Hum Psychopharmacol. 2010;25(6):448–61.
23. Kennedy DO et al. Improved cognitive performance and mental fatigue following a multi-vitamin and mineral supplement with added guaraná (*Paullinia cupana*). Appetite. 2008;50(2–3):506–13.
24. Kennedy DO et al. Effects of high-dose B vitamin complex with vitamin C and minerals on subjective mood and performance in healthy males. Psychopharmacology (Berl). 2010:1–14.
25. Pipingas A et al. The effects of multivitamin supplementation on mood and general well-being in healthy young adults. a laboratory and at-home mobile phone assessment. Appetite. 2013;69:123–36.
26. Long SJ, Benton D. Effects of vitamin and mineral supplementation on stress, mild psychiatric symptoms, and mood in nonclinical samples: a meta-analysis. Psychosom Med. 2013;75(2):144–53.
27. Alpert JE et al. Nutrition and depression: focus on folate. Nutrition. 2000;16(7–8):544–6.
28. Baldewicz TT et al. Cobalamin level is related to self-reported and clinically rated mood and to syndromal depression in bereaved HIV-1+ and HIV-1- homosexual men. J Psychosom Res. 2000;48(2):177–85.
29. Tolmunen T et al. Dietary folate and depressive symptoms are associated in middle-aged Finnish men. J Nutr. 2003;133(10):3233–6.
30. Tiemeier H et al. Vitamin B12, folate, and homocysteine in depression: the Rotterdam study. Am J Psychiatry. 2002;159(12):2099–101.
31. Bjelland I et al. Folate, vitamin B12, homocysteine, and the MTHFR 677C → T polymorphism in anxiety and depression. the Hordaland Homocysteine Study. Arch Gen Psychiatry. 2003;60(6):618–26.
32. Botez MI et al. Folate deficiency and decreased brain 5-hydroxytryptamine synthesis in man and rat [21]. Nature. 1979;278(5700):182–3.
33. Godfrey PSA et al. Enhancement of recovery from psychiatric illness by methylfolate. Lancet. 1990;336(8712):392–5.

34. Passen M et al. Oral 5′-methyltetrahydrofolic acid in senile organic mental disorders with depression: results of a double-blind multicenter study. Aging Clin Exp Res. 1993;5(1):63–71.
35. Coppen A, Bailey J. Enhancement of the antidepressant action of fluoxetine by folic acid: a randomised, placebo controlled trial. J Affect Disord. 2000;60(2):121–30.
36. Alpert JE et al. Folinic acid (leucovorin) as an adjunctive treatment for SSRI-refractory depression. Ann Clin Psychiatry. 2002;14(1):33–8.
37. Taylor MJ et al. Folate for depressive disorders: systematic review and meta-analysis of randomized controlled trials. J Psychopharmacol. 2004;18(2):251–6.
38. Coppen A, Bolander-Gouaille C. Treatment of depression: time to consider folic acid and vitamin B 12. J Psychopharmacol. 2005;19(1):59–65.
39. Rucklidge JJ et al. Shaken but unstirred? Effects of micronutrients on stress and trauma after an earthquake: RCT evidence comparing formulas and doses. Hum Psychopharmacol. 2012;27(5):440–54.
40. Rucklidge JJ et al. Psychological functioning 1 year after a brief intervention using micronutrients to treat stress and anxiety related to the 2011 Christchurch earthquakes: a naturalistic follow-up. Hum Psychopharmacol. 2014;29(3):230–43.
41. Swaminathan R. Magnesium metabolism and its disorders. Clin Biochem Rev. 2003;24(2):47–66.
42. Ford ES, Mokdad AH. Dietary magnesium intake in a national sample of U.S. adults. J Nutr. 2003;133(9):2879–82.
43. Elin RJ. Magnesium metabolism in health and disease. Dis Mon. 1988;34(4):166–218.
44. Mori H et al. Identification by mutagenesis of a Mg2+ – block site of the NMDA receptor channel. Nature. 1992;358(6388):673–5.
45. Decollogne S et al. NMDA receptor complex blockade by oral administration of magnesium: comparison with MK-801. Pharmacol Biochem Behav. 1997;58(1):261–8.
46. Poleszak E et al. Antidepressant- and anxiolytic-like activity of magnesium in mice. Pharmacol Biochem Behav. 2004;78(1):7–12.
47. Eby GA, Eby KL. Rapid recovery from major depression using magnesium treatment. Med Hypotheses. 2006;67(2):362–70.
48. Szewczyk B et al. Antidepressant activity of zinc and magnesium in view of the current hypotheses of antidepressant action. Pharmacol Rep. 2008;60(5):588–99.
49. Frizel D, Coppen A, Marks V. Plasma magnesium and calcium in depression. Br J Psychiatry. 1969;115(529):1375–7.
50. Wacker WE, Parisi AF. Magnesium metabolism. N Engl J Med. 1968;278(12):658–63.
51. Eby Iii GA, Eby KL. Magnesium for treatment-resistant depression: a review and hypothesis. Med Hypotheses. 2010;74(4):649–60.
52. Abraham GE. Nutritional factors in the etiology of the premenstrual tension syndromes. J Reprod Med. 1983;28(7):446–64.
53. De Souza MC et al. A synergistic effect of a daily supplement for 1 month of 200 mg magnesium plus 50 mg vitamin B6 for the relief of anxiety-related premenstrual symptoms: a randomized, double-blind, crossover study. J Womens Health Gend Based Med. 2000;9(2):131–9.
54. Walker AF et al. Magnesium supplementation alleviates premenstrual symptoms of fluid retention. J Womens Health. 1998;7(9):1157–65.
55. Hanus M, Lafon J, Mathieu M. Double-blind, randomised, placebo-controlled study to evaluate the efficacy and safety of a fixed combination containing two plant extracts (*Crataegus oxyacantha* and Eschscholtzia californica) and magnesium in mild-to-moderate anxiety disorders. Curr Med Res Opin. 2004;20(1):63–71.
56. Lakhan SE, Vieira KF. Nutritional and herbal supplements for anxiety and anxiety-related disorders: systematic review. Nutr J. 2010;9(1).
57. Nieves Jr C, Langkamp-Henken B. Arginine and immunity: a unique perspective. Biomed Pharmacother. 2002;56(10):471–82.

58. Smriga M, Torii K. L-Lysine acts like a partial serotonin receptor 4 antagonist and inhibits serotonin-mediated intestinal pathologies and anxiety in rats. Proc Natl Acad Sci U S A. 2003;100(26):15370–5.
59. Chang YF et al. Chronic L-lysine develops anti-pentylenetetrazol tolerance and reduces synaptic GABAergic sensitivity. Eur J Pharmacol. 1993;233(2–3):209–17.
60. Masood A et al. Modulation of stress-induced neurobehavioral changes by nitric oxide in rats. Eur J Pharmacol. 2003;458(1–2):135–9.
61. Srinongkote S et al. A diet fortified with L-lysine and L-arginine reduces plasma cortisol and blocks anxiogenic response to transportation in pigs. Nutr Neurosci. 2003;6(5):283–9.
62. Jezova D et al. Subchronic treatment with amino acid mixture of L-lysine and L-arginine modifies neuroendocrine activation during psychological stress in subjects with high trait anxiety. Nutr Neurosci. 2005;8(3):155–60.
63. Smriga M et al. Oral treatment with L-lysine and L-arginine reduces anxiety and basal cortisol levels in healthy humans. Biomed Res. 2007;28(2):85–90.
64. Smriga M et al. Lysine fortification reduces anxiety and lessens stress in family members in economically weak communities in Northwest Syria. Proc Natl Acad Sci U S A. 2004;101(22):8285–8.
65. Clements Jr RS, Darnell B. Myo-inositol content of common foods: development of a high-myo-inositol diet. Am J Clin Nutr. 1980;33(9):1954–67.
66. Einat H, Belmaker RH. The effects of inositol treatment in animal models of psychiatric disorders. J Affect Disord. 2001;62(1–2):113–21.
67. Frey R et al. Myo-inositol in depressive and healthy subjects determined by frontal 1H-magnetic resonance spectroscopy at 1.5 tesla. J Psychiatr Res. 1998;32(6):411–20.
68. Levine J et al. Inositol treatment raises CSF inositol levels. Brain Res. 1993;627(1):168–70.
69. Rahman S, Neuman RS. Myo-inositol reduces serotonin (5-HT2) receptor induced homologous and heterologous desensitization. Brain Res. 1993;631(2):349–51.
70. Marazziti D et al. Decreased inhibitory activity of PKC in OCD patients after six months of treatment. Psychoneuroendocrinology. 2002;27(7):769–76.
71. Marazziti D et al. Increased inhibitory activity of protein kinase C on the serotonin transporter in OCD. Neuropsychobiology. 2000;41(4):171–7.
72. Einat H et al. The antidepressant activity of inositol in the forced swim test involves 5-HT2 receptors. Behav Brain Res. 2001;118(1):77–83.
73. Harvey BH et al. Defining the neuromolecular action of myo-inositol: application to obsessive-compulsive disorder. Prog Neuropsychopharmacol Biol Psychiatry. 2002;26(1):21–32.
74. Levine J et al. Combination of inositol and serotonin reuptake inhibitors in the treatment of depression. Biol Psychiatry. 1999;45(3):270–3.
75. Camfield DA, Sarris J, Berk M. Nutraceuticals in the treatment of obsessive compulsive disorder (OCD): a review of mechanistic and clinical evidence. Prog Neuropsychopharmacol Biol Psychiatry. 2011;35(4):887–95.
76. Levine J. Controlled trials of inositol in psychiatry. Eur Neuropsychopharmacol. 1997;7(2):147–55.
77. Carey PD et al. Single photon emission computed tomography (SPECT) in obsessive-compulsive disorder before and after treatment with inositol. Metab Brain Dis. 2004;19(1–2):125–34.
78. Levine J, Pomerantz T, Belmaker RH. The effect of inositol on cognitive processes and mood states in normal volunteers. Eur Neuropsychopharmacol. 1994;4(3):417.
79. Mukai T et al. A meta-analysis of inositol for depression and anxiety disorders. Hum Psychopharmacol. 2014;29(1):55–63.
80. Benjamin J et al. Double-blind, placebo-controlled, crossover trial of inositol treatment for panic disorder. Am J Psychiatry. 1995;152(7):1084–6.

81. Benjamin J et al. Acute inositol does not attenuate m-CPP-induced anxiety, mydriasis and endocrine effects in panic disorder. J Psychiatr Res. 1997;31(4):489–95.
82. Kaplan Z et al. Inositol treatment of post-traumatic stress disorder. Anxiety. 1996;2(1):51–2.
83. Fux M et al. Inositol treatment of obsessive-compulsive disorder. Am J Psychiatry. 1996;153(9):1219–21.
84. Fux M, Benjamin J, Belmaker RH. Inositol versus placebo aumentation of serotonin reuptake inhibitor in the treatment of obsessive-compulsive disorder: a double-blind cross-over study. Int J Neuropsychopharmacol. 1999;2(3):193–5.
85. Seedat S, Stein DJ. Inositol augmentation of serotonin reuptake inhibitors in treatment-refractory obsessive – compulsive disorder: an open trial. Int Clin Psychopharmacol. 1999;14(6):353–6.
86. Seedat S, Stein DJ, Harvey BH. Inositol in the treatment of trichotillomania and compulsive skin picking [5]. J Clin Psychiatry. 2001;62(1):60–1.
87. Levine J et al. Double-blind, controlled trial of inositol treatment of depression. Am J Psychiatry. 1995;152(5):792–4.
88. Bonanomi L, Gazzaniga A. Toxicology, pharmacokinetics and metabolism of acetylcysteine. Eur J Respir Dis Suppl. 1980;111:45–51.
89. Pendyala L, Creaven PJ. Pharmacokinetic and pharmacodynamic studies of N-acetylcysteine, a potential chemopreventive agent during a Phase I trial. Cancer Epidemiol Biomarkers and Prev. 1995;4(3):245–51.
90. Allegra L et al. Human neutrophil oxidative bursts and their in vitro modulation by different N-acetylcysteine concentrations. Arzneimittelforschung. 2002;52(9):669–76.
91. Atkuri KR, Mantovani JJ, Herzenberg LA. N-Acetylcysteine-a safe antidote for cysteine/glutathione deficiency. Curr Opin Pharmacol. 2007;7(4):355–9.
92. Samuni Y et al. The chemistry and biological activities of N-acetylcysteine. Biochim Biophys Acta. 2013;1830(8):4117–29.
93. Katz M et al. Cerebrospinal fluid concentrations of N-acetylcysteine after oral administration in Parkinson's disease. Parkinsonism Relat Disord. 2015;21(5):500–3.
94. Pittenger C, Bloch MH, Williams K. Glutamate abnormalities in obsessive compulsive disorder: neurobiology, pathophysiology, and treatment. Pharmacol Ther. 2011;132(3):314–32.
95. Berk M et al. Glutathione: a novel treatment target in psychiatry. Trends Pharmacol Sci. 2008;29(7):346–51.
96. Camfield DA. The actions of N-Acetylcysteine in the central nervous system: Implications for the treatment of neurodegenerative and neuropsychiatric disorders. In: Scholey AB, Stough C, editors. Advances in natural medicines, nutraceuticals and neurocognition. Florida: CRC Press, Taylor & Francis Group; 2013.
97. Costa-Campos L et al. Interactive effects of N-acetylcysteine and antidepressants. Prog Neuropsychopharmacol Biol Psychiatry. 2013;44:125–30.
98. De Rosa SC et al. N-acetylcysteine replenishes glutathione in HIV infection. Eur J Clin Invest. 2000;30(10):915–29.
99. Deepmala et al. Clinical trials of N-acetylcysteine in psychiatry and neurology: a systematic review. Neurosci Biobehav Rev. 2015;55:294–321.
100. Berk M et al. The promise of N-acetylcysteine in neuropsychiatry. Trends Pharmacol Sci. 2013;34(3):167–77.
101. Strawn JR, Saldaña SN. Treatment with adjunctive N-acetylcysteine in an adolescent with selective serotonin reuptake inhibitor-resistant anxiety. J Child Adolesc Psychopharmacol. 2012;22(6):472–3.
102. Behl A et al. Relationship of possible stress-related biochemical markers to oxidative/antioxidative status in obsessive-compulsive disorder. Neuropsychobiology. 2010;61(4):210–4.
103. Ozdemir E et al. Serum selenium and plasma malondialdehyde levels and antioxidant enzyme activities in patients with obsessive-compulsive disorder. Prog Neuropsychopharmacol Biol Psychiatry. 2009;33(1):62–5.

104. Konuk N et al. Plasma levels of tumor necrosis factor-alpha and interleukin-6 in obsessive compulsive disorder. Mediators Inflamm. 2007;2007.
105. Ng F et al. Oxidative stress in psychiatric disorders: evidence base and therapeutic implications. Int J Neuropsychopharmacol. 2008;11(6):851–76.
106. Lafleur DL et al. N-acetylcysteine augmentation in serotonin reuptake inhibitor refractory obsessive-compulsive disorder. Psychopharmacology (Berl). 2006;184(2):254–6.
107. Van Ameringen M et al. N-acetylcysteine augmentation in treatment resistant obsessive compulsive disorder: a case series. J Obesessive-Compuls Relat Disord. 2013;2(1):48–52.
108. Afshar H et al. N-acetylcysteine add-on treatment in refractory obsessive-compulsive disorder: a randomized, double-blind, placebo-controlled trial. J Clin Psychopharmacol. 2012;32(6):797–803.
109. Sarris J et al. N-Acetyl Cysteine (NAC) in the treatment of obsessive-compulsive disorder: a 16-week, double-blind, randomised, placebo-controlled study. CNS Drugs. 2015;29(9):801–9.
110. Sarris, J., et al. Participant characteristics as modifiers of response to N-Acetyl cysteine (NAC) in Obsessive-Compulsive Disorder. Clin Psychol Sci. http://dx.doi.org/10.1177/2167702616639864.
111. Berk M et al. Nail-biting stuff? The effect of N-acetyl cysteine on nail-biting. CNS Spectr. 2009;14(7):357–60.
112. Ghanizadeh A, Derakhshan N, Berk M. N-acetylcysteine versus placebo for treating nail biting, a double blind randomized placebo controlled clinical trial. Anti-Inflamm Antiallergy Agents Med Chem. 2013;12(3):223–8.
113. Grant JE, Odlaug BL, Suck WK. N-acetylcysteine, a glutamate modulator, in the treatment of trichotillomania: a double-blind, placebo-controlled study. Arch Gen Psychiatry. 2009;66(7):756–63.
114. Odlaug BL, Grant JE. N-acetyl cysteine in the treatment of grooming disorders. J Clin Psychopharmacol. 2007;27(2):227–9.
115. Rodrigues-Barata AR et al. N-acetylcysteine in the treatment of trichotillomania. Int J Trichol. 2012;4(3):176–8.
116. Silva-Netto R et al. N-acetylcysteine in the treatment of skin-picking disorder. Rev Bras Psiquiatr. 2014;36(1):101.
117. Oliver G et al. N-acetyl cysteine in the treatment of obsessive compulsive and related disorders: a systematic review. Clin Psychopharmacol Neurosci. 2015;13(1):12–24.
118. Firoz M, Graber M. Bioavallability of US commercial magnesium preparations. Magnes Res. 2001;14(4):257–62.
119. Lindberg JS et al. Magnesium bioavailability from magnesium citrate and magnesium oxide. J Am Coll Nutr. 1990;9(1):48–55.
120. Walker AF et al. Mg citrate found more bioavailable than other Mg preparations in a randomised, double-blind study. Magnes Res. 2003;16(3):183–91.
121. Böger RH, Bode-Böger SM. The clinical pharmacology of L-arginine. Annu Rev Pharmacol Toxicol. 2001:79–99.
122. L-arginine. Review of natural products. Facts & comparisons [database online]. October 2010, St. Louis: Wolters Kluwer Health Inc.
123. Carlomagno G et al. Myo-inositol in the treatment of premenstrual dysphoric disorder. Hum Psychopharmacol. 2011;26(7):526–30.

6 Treatments for Comorbid Anxiety and Mood Disorders

Jerome Sarris and David Mischoulon

6.1 Introduction

Anxiety disorders (such as generalized anxiety disorder) are highly comorbid with depression [1–3], and the polyvalent effects from herbal medicines can potentially target a range of symptoms that commonly overlap in these disorders. Herbal medicines with mood-elevating effects may also have anxiolytic effects. This may be due to modulation of neurological pathways that have both antidepressant and anxiolytic effects (in particular, the GABA and serotonin systems), or this may be due to anxiety being reduced when depression is adequately treated [4, 5]. For example, this effect was found in the case of a recent double-blind, randomized controlled trial (RCT) involving participants with generalized anxiety, which found that while *Piper methysticum* (kava) significantly reduced participants' anxiety beyond placebo, this also occurred for their depression levels [6]. Various nutraceuticals have been shown to provide antidepressant activity, with several having notable antidepressant effects: *Hypericum perforatum* (St John's wort), *Crocus sativus* (saffron), omega-3 fatty acids, S-adenosyl methionine (SAMe), and zinc [7]. These may have a prescriptive role in treating depression co-occurring with anxiety, though it should be noted that none of these agents have been shown to have primary anxiolytic effects.

J. Sarris (✉)
University of Melbourne, Department of Psychiatry, The Melbourne Clinic, The Professorial Unit, ARCADIA Mental Health Research Group, 2 Salisbury St, Richmond, Melbourne, VIC 3121, Australia

Centre for Human Psychopharmacology, Swinburne University of Technology, Hawthorn, VIC, Australia
e-mail: jsarris@unimelb.edu.au

D. Mischoulon
Depression Clinical and Research Program, Department of Psychiatry, Massachusetts General Hospital, Harvard Medical School, Boston, MA, USA

D. Camfield et al. (eds.), *Evidence-Based Herbal and Nutritional Treatments for Anxiety in Psychiatric Disorders*, DOI 10.1007/978-3-319-42307-4_6

6.2 St John's Wort (*Hypericum perforatum*)

6.2.1 Overview

Hypericum perforatum (St John's wort: SJW) has been used for millennia for a range of nervous system conditions, including depression [8]. While dozens of clinical trials have consistently demonstrated SJW's efficacy in improving mood, after two RCTs a decade ago revealed no greater efficacy than placebo [9, 10], clinical regard for the nutraceutical lessened. Notably, the negative results in those studies did not reveal a lack of antidepressant efficacy per se, but rather reflected a pattern of increasing placebo-response (and decreasing effect sizes), which also exists with conventional antidepressant studies for mild to moderate depression [11, 12]. While an abundance of SJW depression studies have been conducted, a paucity of research exists on its clinical applications in other psychiatric disorders, in particular anxiety disorders.

6.2.2 Mechanisms of Action

6.2.2.1 Constituents

SJW contains an abundance of constituents. These include the napthodianthrones hypericin and pseudohypericin; in addition to the phloroglucinol compound hyperforin; and a range of flavonoids, volatile oils, and tannins [13]. Antidepressant in vitro and in vivo research has demonstrated a range of neurobiological activities, including: nonselective inhibition of the neuronal reuptake of serotonin, noradrenalin, and dopamine, in addition to weak monoamine oxidase A and B inhibition [14]. Other biological effects include decreased degradation of neurochemicals, and sensitization of/and increased binding of ligands to various receptors (e.g., glutamate, GABA, and adenosine), increased dopaminergic activity in the prefrontal cortex in animal models, and neuroendocrine modulation [8]. It should be noted that the biological effects revealed in many preclinical studies have used exceedingly high doses of SJW or its isolated constituents (far in excess of typically clinical doses). Further, the poor bioavailability of many constituents, and the lack of penetration across the blood–brain barrier (particularly from hypericin) [15] indicate that caution needs to be applied when extrapolating from preclinical studies to human clinical activity. The pharmacokinetics vary between active constituents. The half-life of hypericin has been documented as~21 h, with the peak serum level occurring after ~6 h; hyperforin has a half-life of~9 h, and time to peak plasma of~3.5 h; while the different flavonoid compounds vary with half-lives ranging from 1 to 9 h [16–18]. The common daily dosage of concentrated SJW is between 900 and 1800 mg (depending on standardization). This is often given in two to three doses per day in tablet form, being standardized to about 0.3 % of hypericin and/or 1–5 % of hyperforin.

6.2.3 Evidence of Efficacy

6.2.3.1 Depression

To date, over 40 clinical trials of varying methodological quality have been conducted assessing the efficacy of SJW in treating depressed mood. A meta-analysis of RCTs involving SJW for depression by Linde and colleagues [19] revealed a Relative Risk [RR] of 1.48 (1.23, 1.77) from 18 combined studies for response of SJW versus placebo, and an equivocal effect to selective serotonin reuptake inhibitors (SSRIs) of 1.00 (0.90, 1.15). Another later meta-analysis conducted by Rahimi and colleagues [20] found a significant RR for response of 1.22 (1.03, 1.45) in favor of SJW over placebo, with a small weighted mean difference between treatments of 1.33 points (1.15, 1.51) on the Hamilton Depression Rating Scale (HAMD). Comparison with SSRIs yielded a nonsignificant difference between treatments of 0.32 (−1.28, 0.64) for mean reduction of HAMD score from baseline. It should be noted that most of the extracts analyzed in the meta-analysis were standardized European formulas such as LI-160, Ze-117, or WS-5570.

6.2.3.2 Anxiety and Other Psychiatric Disorders

Apart from application in depression, SJW has been studied in social phobia, obsessive-compulsive disorder (OCD), somatoform disorders, and attention-deficit hyperactivity disorder (ADHD). While anecdotally SJW has been recommended for anxiety, there is no research-based evidence supporting this application. For use in OCD, an open-label study [21] initially indicated that SJW was a promising intervention for this disorder; however, a more recent controlled study did not support this finding. This RCT recruited 60 participants with a primary diagnosis of OCD to 12 weeks of randomized treatment of SJW or placebo (flexible dosing of LI 160; 600–1800 mg depending on response) [22]. Results revealed that the mean reduction on the Yale-Brown Obsessive Compulsive Scale (Y-BOCS) in the active group did not differ significantly compared to the placebo group. In social phobia, one pilot RCT testing SJW (flexible-dose 600–1800 mg daily) also found no significant differential benefit over placebo [23].

Two RCTs using SJW to treat somatoform disorders have been conducted. A 6-week multicenter RCT involving 151 patients with ICD-10 diagnosed somatization or somatoform disorder, found that SJW LI 160 extract (600 mg per day) was superior to placebo in reducing somatoform symptoms [24]. Another 6-week RCT trialed the LI 160 SJW extract in 184 patients with somatization disorders, and found that 45.4 % of the SJW group were classified as responders (compared with 20.9 % who took placebo) [25]. ADHD is highly comorbid with anxiety disorders and it shares some of these neurobiological dysfunctions [26–28]. An 8-week RCT investigating 900 mg daily of standardized SJW or matched placebo in the treatment of 54 children/adolescents with ADHD [29] revealed no significant difference between SJW and placebo on the ADHD Rating Scale-IV. Nor was any effect found on any attention or hyperactivity subscale.

6.3 Saffron (*Crocus sativus*)

6.3.1 Overview

Saffron is a lucrative commodity native to Western Asia. It has been used in traditional medicine to treat a range of health conditions, including mood disorders, muscular spasms, menstrual disorders, and general pain [30]. Different preparations of saffron, including its stigma and its petals have been used clinically, with the stigma being more preferable (although more expensive). The active constituents involved in therapeutic activity of Saffron stigma include an estimated 40–50 major constituents. High-quality saffron contains approximately 30 % crocins, 5–15 % picrocrocin, and over 5 % volatile compounds including safranal [30].

6.3.2 Mechanisms of Action

Animal models using ethanolic extracts of saffron and its constituents safranal and crocin, have shown antidepressant, anxiolytic, and hypnotic effects [31]. Crocin's antidepressant activity is purported to occur via re-uptake inhibition of norepinephrine and dopamine, and safranal via serotonin reuptake inhibition [30]. In vitro, crocin has been found to have a weak, but significant affinity for the N-methyl-D-aspartate receptor, reducing ethanol-induced depression [32], in addition to having GABA(A) modulating activity [33, 34]. Administration of saffron and its active constituent crocin have protected against stress-induced impairment of learning and memory, as well as reducing oxidative stress damage to the hippocampus [35]. The constituents of saffron have also shown pronounced antioxidant and neuroprotective activity to attenuate cerebral ischemia-induced oxidative damage, and provide immunomodulatory effects (including anti-inflammatory effects) in rat brain microglial cells [36, 37].

6.3.3 Evidence of Efficacy

Two double-blind RCTs using 30 mg of concentrated saffron extract have demonstrated significant improvement of DSM-IV diagnosed depression over placebo on the HAMD [38, 39]. The Akhondzadeh and colleagues [38] RCT (n = 40) using 30 mg/day of saffron stigma had a large effect size of d = 1.51, while the Moshiri and colleagues [39] RCT (n = 40), which used 30 mg/day of the less expensive saffron petals (as opposed to stigma), revealed a similarly large effect size d = 1.78. In three double-blind RCTs comparing the herbal medicine to imipramine and fluoxetine for major depressive disorder, an equivalent effect was revealed [40–42]. For example, in a study of saffron petals (30 mg/day) versus fluoxetine in the treatment of mild to moderate depression, a 6-week double-blind RCT found the plant medicine to have similar efficacy to fluoxetine (p = 0.71), with no significant adverse effects [41]. Another 6-week RCT using saffron in forty adults with mild to moderate depression, found that saffron stigma (30 mg/day) affected a 12-point significant reduction on the HAMD over placebo (<0.001) [38]. There were no significant differences in the two groups in terms of the observed side effects. It should be noted that while these results are encouraging, larger studies in other countries (besides Iran) are advised.

6.4 Omega-3 Polyunsaturated Fatty Acids

6.4.1 Overview

Over the past century, Western society as a whole has been consuming less omega-3 fatty acids (*n*-3FAs), while increasing dietary omega-6 (*n*-6), as typically found in processed foods rich in vegetable oils [43]. Consequently, individuals who live in Western countries have a higher physiologic ratio of *n*-6:*n*-3 fatty acids than their counterparts in countries with higher fish and *n*-3 consumption [43]. Stress has also, in combination with dietary practices, been suggested to promote a proinflammatory state in humans, which may contribute to cardiovascular and psychiatric illness [43]. Administration of *n*-3FA supplements may potentially correct the *n*-6FA:*n*-3FA ratio, thus reversing a proinflammatory state and providing beneficial cardiovascular and psychiatric effects [44]. There has been much research conducted over the past two decades to examine the role of *n*-3FAs in psychiatry. Evidence from treatment studies generally supports clinical efficacy in unipolar depression and bipolar disorder, and possible milder benefits in psychotic and personality disorders. Eicosapentaenoic acid (EPA; 20:5) and the longer chain docosahexaenoic acid (DHA; 22:6), both of which are found primarily in fish oil and other marine sources, are the *n*-3FAs most commonly used in psychiatric populations.

6.4.2 Mechanisms of Action

Omega-3 fatty acids have a critical role in neural function, and have great potential for treating depression, especially if an inflammatory causation is present [45, 46]. The antidepressant activity of *n*-3FAs appears to occur via modulation of norepinephrine, dopamine and serotonin reuptake, degradation, synthesis, and receptor binding; anti-inflammatory effects; and the enhancement of cell membrane fluidity via being incorporated into membrane walls [47]. Specific mood-related mechanisms of *n*-3FAs may include an effect on membrane-bound receptors and enzymes that regulate neurotransmitter signaling, as well as regulation of calcium ion influx through calcium channels [48]. These mechanisms may help stabilize neuronal membranes and promote their fluidity. For example, administration of EPA plus DHA to healthy subjects lowered their plasma norepinephrine levels compared with placebo, suggesting that *n*-3FAs interact with catecholamines [49]. Regarding inflammatory pathways, *n*-3FA administration may inhibit secretion of inflammatory cytokines by opposing *n*-6FA-derived eicosanoids, thus attenuating corticosteroid release from the adrenal gland and dampening cortisol-related mood-altering effects [48].

6.4.3 Evidence of Efficacy

n-3FAs have been studied largely as a treatment for mood disorders, as well as for a few other conditions such as schizophrenia and personality disorders. At this time, there are more than 35 published controlled trials and a few open studies using EPA monotherapy or a combination of EPA and DHA at doses representing at least five times the usual Western dietary intake (which is usually suboptimal). By and large, these studies support antidepressant and/or mood-stabilizing effects. There are few data regarding efficacy of DHA alone; however, no RCTs to date have shown a beneficial effect. While several reviews and meta-analyses of *n*-3FAs generally support their efficacy in depressed populations [50], the body of work is noted for small samples, heterogeneity involving both augmentation and monotherapy, as well as mixing unipolar and bipolar subjects, and a broad range of *n*-3 doses (from 1 to 10 g/d) and EPA:DHA ratios [51]. In fact, statistical significance and effect sizes of at least moderate strength (0.41 [95 % CI: 0.26, 0.55]) were only evident in more severe levels of depression, or for trials that enrolled individuals with a diagnosed depressive disorder. While not all monotherapy studies support *n*-3FAs for depression, the strongest evidence exists for adjunctive use with SSRIs [52]. A recent meta-analysis of six bipolar disorder studies found a significant but moderate effect in favor of *n*-3FAs (Hedges $g = 0.34$; $p = 0.029$) for bipolar depression [47], and a nonsignificant trend in favor of *n*-3FAs (Hedges $g = 0.20$; $p = 0.099$) for mania. Thus, most of the benefit from *n*-3FAs in bipolar subjects appears to be for the depressive rather than manic phase of the illness.

With regard to the evaluation of efficacy for EPA in comparison to DHA, meta-analyses by Martins [53] and Sublette and colleagues (2011) found that EPA preparations, or those with higher proportion or EPA relative to DHA, potentially have a stronger antidepressant effect than for DHA alone. The meta-analytic comparison between DHA and EPA found that DHA monotherapy was not significant, whereas studies using supplements containing >50 % EPA had a significant antidepressant effect ($p = 0.005$) [45]. Not all research supports this however, as evidenced by a recent 8-week, double-blind RCT involving 196 adults with DSM-IV MDD and a baseline HAMD-17 score ≥ 15 who were prescribed EPA-enriched *n*-3 1000 mg/d versus DHA-enriched *n*-3 1000 mg/d, or placebo [54]. All three treatment groups demonstrated statistically significant improvement in reduction of depression scores, and thus EPA was not shown to be significantly better than placebo or DHA. While this study could not rule out placebo effects as a contributor to *n*-3FAs' antidepressant effect, an ancillary investigation suggested that baseline inflammation may be a determinant of response to *n*-3FAs. A subanalysis of this study found that while overall treatment group differences were negligible, participants with any "'high" baseline inflammatory biomarkers (IL-1ra or hs-CRP) improved more on EPA than placebo or DHA and less on DHA [44].

6.5 SAMe (*S-Adenosyl methionine*)

6.5.1 Overview

SAMe has gained much popularity in the United States since it was marketed as an over-the-counter dietary supplement in the late 1990s. Because it has a broad range of activity, SAMe has been used to treat various medical conditions (including arthritis and liver conditions), and in particular for improving mood. SAMe is a major methyl donor in the brain, contributing to synthesis of hormones, neurotransmitters, nucleic acids, proteins, and phospholipids [55]. SAMe is synthesized from the amino acid l-methionine through the one-carbon cycle, a metabolic pathway that includes folate and B12 [55]. Deficiencies of folate and B12 have been linked to depression. Vitamin B12 is converted to methylcobalamin, which also plays a role in neurotransmitter synthesis, but there is little if any evidence for antidepressant efficacy of B12 supplementation. On the other hand, between 10–30 % of depressed patients may have low folate, which may dampen antidepressant response [56], and augmentation of antidepressants with various folate forms may have beneficial effects on mood [57, 58]. The mood-enhancing effects of folate and/or B12 may be executed via downstream increases in SAMe levels.

6.5.2 Mechanisms of Action

SAMe is an endogenous sulfur-containing compound that, as discussed above, is a critical neurochemical component involved in the one-carbon cycle responsible for the methylation of neurotransmitters that regulate mood [59, 60]. SAMe may improve depressed mood via enhanced methylation of catecholamines and increased serotonin turnover, reuptake inhibition of norepinephrine, enhanced dopaminergic activity, decreased prolactin secretion, and increased phosphatidylcholine conversion [55]. Animal depression models have also shown SAMe to restore the levels of putrescine in the nucleus accumbens [61]; this polyamine being shown to have antidepressant effects [62].

6.5.3 Evidence of Efficacy

SAMe has strong evidence as an antidepressant agent, with double-blind studies demonstrating that parenteral or oral preparations of SAMe, compared with a number of standard tricyclic antidepressants such as clomipramine, amitriptyline, and imipramine, are generally equally effective, and tend to produce fewer side effects [55]. Among eight well-designed placebo-controlled studies with sample sizes ranging from 40 to100 and doses ranging from 200 to 1600 mg/day (PO, IM, IV), SAMe demonstrated superiority to placebo in six of them, and equivalency in two [55]. SAMe has been shown in some cases to have a faster onset of action than conventional antidepressants. One study of injected SAMe augmentation of imipramine reported that patients improved within a few days compared to imipramine plus adjunctive placebo (although this statistical difference diminished after 2 weeks) [63]. SAMe may be an effective adjunctive treatment for depression, with an RCT revealing that SAMe augmentation in 73 MDD participants who were partial and nonresponders to SSRIs and SNRIs was more effective in reducing depression than placebo [64].

Not all research, however, is in favor of SAMe. A recently reported double-blind RCT comparing the efficacy of SAMe versus placebo and a standard SSRI (escitalopram) in treating MDD, found that the 12-week two-site study was essentially negative, with no significant differences in clinical response occurring between the three treatment groups [65]. A subanalysis of data from one of the study sites, which recruited the majority of participants, revealed however a significant effect in favor of SAMe, with a moderate-to-large effect size versus placebo ($d = 0.74$) [66]. Remission rates were also significantly higher for SAMe (34 %) than for escitalopram (23 %) or placebo (6 %). Further analysis revealed that there was a gender difference between the sites (59 % males in site 1; and 31 % males in site 2; $X^2 p < 0.0001$), and that in fact significant reduction of depression was seen only in males for combined sites between treatments from baseline to study endpoint (a 4.3-point difference between males and females, $p = 0.034$) [67].

6.5.3.1 Other Psychiatric Conditions

Other reports suggest that SAMe is effective for cognitive deficits seen in dementia. Reduced folate and B12, as well as decreased membrane fluidity have been found in patients with Alzheimer's disease [68]. Other studies have suggested that SAMe may treat pregnancy-related cholestasis (impaired bile flow) and relieve distress during the purpuerium [69]. SAMe has also been shown to reduce psychological distress during opioid detoxification, and may be effective in dual diagnosis patients with depression and alcoholism or drug addiction [70]. At least two studies suggest effectiveness at doses ranging from 800 to 3600 mg/day for depressed patients with Parkinson's disease [71, 72]. Because of its good tolerability and low risk of interactions, SAMe may be generally useful in medically ill depressed patients for whom a reduction in the risk of adverse effects from conventional antidepressants is desired [70].

6.6 Zinc

6.6.1 Overview

The mineral zinc is a divalent cation that is one of the most prevalent trace elements in the amygdala, hippocampus, and neocortex, and is involved with a range of crucial neurochemical processes [73, 74]. Zinc is an essential element that is involved in many enzymatic reactions, and is also vital for normal human development, wound healing, and immune function [75]. As the body cannot store zinc, a steady state is required via nutrition or supplementation.

6.6.2 Mechanisms of Action

Zinc is involved with hippocampal neurogenesis via its effects on the upregulation of brain-derived neurotrophic factor (BDNF), while also modifying N-methyl-D-aspartate (NMDA) and glutamate activity [74]. Zinc modulates the hypothalmic-pituitary adrenal axis, and has been shown to be neuroprotective in animal models. Low zinc serum level is associated with depression risk, and correlated with an increase in the activation immune system biomarkers, suggesting that this effect may result in part from a depression-related alteration in the immune-inflammatory system [76]. Zinc supplementation has been found to attenuate inflammation via inhibition of TNF-alpha, and IL-1beta [75].

6.6.3 Evidence of Efficacy

A meta-analysis comparing peripheral blood zinc concentrations between depressed and nondepressed participants included 17 studies and revealed zinc concentrations were approximately −1.85 micromol/L lower in depressed participants compared to control subjects (CI 95 %:−2.51 to −1.19 μmol/L, $p < 0.001$) [77]. Greater depression severity was associated with greater relative zinc deficiency. An example is reflected in a cross-sectional study that examined the relationship between dietary intake of zinc and depression in 402 postgraduate students [76]. Results revealed an inverse relationship between dietary intake of zinc and depression. The results persisted after being controlled for several potential confounding variables related to depressive symptoms, for example, sex, years of education, smoking status.

A review by Lai and colleagues [78] regarding all published RCTs of zinc and depression found four studies that met inclusion criteria. Two key 12-week RCTs that examined the effects of zinc (25 mg/d) monotherapy supplementation as an adjunct to antidepressants, such as SSRIs, found that the mineral significantly lowered depressive symptom scores of depressed patients (pooled standard mean difference over placebo on HAMD of −2.84 points, $p < 0.001$). Interestingly, subtherapeutic doses of zinc have also been shown in animal depression models to elicit a synergistic effect in enhancing the antidepressant activity of several antidepressants [79]. This combined evidence suggests potential benefits of zinc as a stand-alone intervention or as an adjunct to conventional antidepressant drug therapy for depression. Amino acid or picolinate forms are advised to be used due to improved absorbability [80].

6.6.4 Clinical Considerations

Given the apparent efficacy, safety, and tolerability of the nutraceuticals detailed in this chapter (Table 6.1), these can be prescribed with confidence by clinicians to treat depressed mood which may co-occur with anxiety. Some safety considerations still need to be identified. First, while research indicates outcome equivalence

Table 6.1 Mood-elevating nutraceuticals

Nutraceutical	Dosage	Major/active constituents	Key evidence	Potential AEs	Potential clinical use	Clinical advice
St John's wort (*Hypericum perforatum*)	1 mg of hypericin per day (one or two times per day); about 900 mg/day of SJW preparation	Hypercin,Hyperforin,Flavonoids	Meta-analyses showing a significant effect in favor of SJW over placebo and equivalence to antidepressants	Serotonin syndrome Switching to mania Skin reactions Digestive upsets	Major depressive disorder Somatoform disorder	Do not co-prescribe with antidepressants; caution with bipolar disorder; avoid high hyperforin extracts if co-medicating; caution regarding interactions with other medications
Saffron	Standardized for 30 mg of crocin and 5 mg of safranal per day	Crocin Safranal	RCTs showing greater antidepressant effect than placebo and equivalence to SSRIs	Tachycardia Sweating Anxiety Insomnia	Depressed mood	Can be expensive; however, petal extracts may also be effective
Omega-3	3–6 capsules per day standardized to approximately 1 g of EPA per day	EPA DHA	Meta-analyses showing an antidepressant effect for EPA-rich extracts. Adjunctive use may have a greater clinical effect	Blood thinning Digestive upsets Loose stools Belching	Major depressive disorder Depressed mood with cardiovascular or inflammatory conditions	A safe and inexpensive treatment. EPA-rich formulas advised. Monitor use with anticoagulants

S-adenosyl methionine	800–1600 mg per day	Usually tosylate form (70 % + of active isomers)	Clinical studies have consistently revealed antidepressant effects	Mania switching Serotonin syndrome	Major Depressive Disorder Sexual Dysfunction from antidepressants	Quality issues, and can be expensive
Zinc	20–30 mg elemental (amino acid or picolinate chelates)	Zinc element	Two adjunctive RCTs showing efficacy in improving mood	Nausea Digestive complaints	Depressionand co-occurring immune dysfunction	Advised to prescribe within dosage recommendations long-term

SJW St John's wort, *RCTs* double-blind randomized controlled trials, *SSRIs* selective serotonin reuptake inhibitors between several nutraceuticals and antidepressants in respect to improving mood, replacing these medications with natural agents is not advised in cases of more severe depression and/or suicidality. *n*-3FAs may be particularly well-suited for pregnant or lactating women, elderly people who may not tolerate side effects of conventional antidepressants, and people with cardiovascular disease or autoimmune conditions, for which there may be dual benefits. Still, upper limits of safe doses have not yet been established in pregnancy and lactation, and so caution is still advised in this population. It appears that EPA or EPA-rich preparations should be recommended preferentially over DHA, with approximately 1 g of EPA per day being effective.

With regard to SAMe, there is fairly strong evidence that oral or intravenous SAMe is effective for treatment of major depression, and may even have a faster onset of action than conventional antidepressants. It may be used as monotherapy or in combination with other antidepressants and anxiolytics, and may even accelerate the effect of conventional antidepressants. SAMe has demonstrated good tolerability, no toxicity, lack of drug–drug interactions, and a relatively benign side-effect profile, with minor gastrointestinal complaints (such as dyspepsia, nausea, or stool changes) or stimulation/agitation being the most commonly reported [65]. It may be especially good for elderly and/or medically ill patients in whom side effects and interactions may be a significant concern. There have been some reports of SAMe causing increased anxiety and mania in bipolar patients with depression [81], so caution needs to be taken with bipolar individuals. SAMe is among the more expensive of psychotropic nutraceuticals (costing approximately US$25–$50 per week based on an 800 mg or 1600 mg daily dose), and the instability of the pure compound requires costly manufacturing procedures (e.g., tosylation) and storage elements (e.g., blister packs). Doses reported in the literature range from 400 to 3200 mg/day, though some individuals may require even higher doses for symptomatic relief. SAMe augmentation of conventional antidepressants in cases of partial response, appears to be a viable niche for this compound.

An overarching issue concerning clinicians prescribing SJW is the marked difference in preparation quality and standardization among products [82]; thus, the results of high-quality European pharmaceutical grade extracts cannot be generalized to inferior extracts. Clinicians are advised to use standardized SJW products (such as LI-160, Ze-117, or WS-5570 extracts) which have proven efficacy in clinical trials, to better ensure replication of results. The common daily dosage of concentrated SJW is 900 mg, often given in two to three doses per day in tablet form, amounting to about 1mcg of hypericin (one active component) and/or 0.5–5 % of hyperforin (depending on whether the extract is standardized to reduce hyperforin). However, more severely depressed patients may need up to 1800 mg/day. If needing to avoid drug interactions, the low hyperforin extract ZE-117 may be advised; however, it should be noted that hyperforin crosses the blood–brain barrier, whereas hypericin does not [15]. SJW has not been studied in treatment-resistant depression, and it is unlikely in many cases to exert a potent enough thymoleptic effect required.

While concerns exist over interactions between SJW and various pharmaceuticals, this issue centers on extracts containing higher amounts of hyperforin, which is responsible for inducing cytochrome (CYP) P450 pathways and the P-glycoprotein drug efflux pump, thereby reducing drug serum levels [83]. For this reason, clinicians are advised to only prescribe low-hyperforin SJW products if the patient is taking other medication. Products standardized for higher levels of hypericin and flavonoids should not induce CYP pathways [84]. While SJW has a sound safety profile, case reports have reported possible SJW-induced mania, psychosis, and serotonin syndrome [8]. While many of these mania cases detail concomitant use of other medications and/or recreational drugs, and a background of cyclothymia, a clear temporal association appears to exist between SJW use and induction of hypomania or mania. Therefore, caution is advised in people with a personal or family history of bipolar disorder. Several case reports of serotonin syndrome have been documented by drug surveillance agencies, and this is likely due to use of high-dose SJW and/or concomitant use with synthetic antidepressants, particularly serotonergic agents. Considering this risk, SJW should not be co-prescribed with antidepressants; although there may a role for low-dose SJW when a patient is withdrawing from an antidepressant, or potentially in pregnancy (with appropriate clinical judgment and supervision).

In respect to saffron, while the stigma is fairly expensive, the less expensive petals have still been found to be effective in MDD. The daily doses of up to 1.5 g have been found to be safe [30], with a "Generally Recognized as Safe" (GRAS) status in the United States [85]. In clinical studies, only rare minor adverse effects have been found, for example, digestive upsets, insomnia, irritability, and tachycardia [30]. A 1-week double-blind RCT in humans evaluated saffron stigma tablets (200–400 mg) for short-term safety and tolerability in 10 healthy adults [86]. Clinical examination showed no gross biological or clinical changes in all volunteers after intervention, with no major adverse events reported during the small pilot trial. Finally, regarding zinc prescription, no major adverse effects should occur. It should, however, be advised for consumers to avoid consumption on an empty stomach (may cause nausea), and not exceeding the recommended dosage to prevent an imbalance between other minerals consumed (due to competitive absorption).

References

1. Kessler RC et al. Co-morbid major depression and generalized anxiety disorders in the National Comorbidity Survey follow-up. Psychol Med. 2008;38(3):365–74.
2. Mellman TA. Sleep and anxiety disorders. Psychiatr Clin North Am. 2006;29(4):1047–58 ; abstract x.
3. Roth T. Insomnia as a risk factor for depression. Int J Neuropsychopharmacol. 2004;7:S34–5.
4. Brady KT, Verduin ML. Pharmacotherapy of comorbid mood, anxiety, and substance use disorders. Subst Use Misuse. 2005;40(13–14):2021–41 ,2043–8.
5. Nierenberg AA. Current perspectives on the diagnosis and treatment of major depressive disorder. Am J Manag Care. 2001;7(Suppl11):S353–66.
6. Sarris J et al. The Kava Anxiety Depression Spectrum Study (KADSS): a randomized, placebo-controlled, cross-over trial using an aqueous extract of *Piper methysticum*. Psychopharmacology (Berl). 2009;205(3):399–407.
7. Sarris J et al. Nutritional medicine as mainstream in psychiatry. Lancet Psychiatry. 2015;2(3):271–4.

8. Sarris J, Kavanagh DJ. Kava and St John's wort: current evidence for use in mood and anxiety disorders. J Altern Complement Med. 2009;15(8):827–36.
9. Hypericum Depression Trial Study Group. Effect of *Hypericum perforatum* (St John's wort) in major depressive disorder: a randomized controlled trial. JAMA. 2002;287(14):1807–14.
10. Shelton RC et al. Effectiveness of St John's wort in major depression: a randomized controlled trial. JAMA. 2001;285(15):1978–86.
11. Fournier J et al. Antidepressant drug effects and depression severity: a patient-level meta-analysis. JAMA. 2010;303(1):47–53.
12. Werneke U, Horn O, Taylor D. How effective is St John's wort? The evidence revisited. J Clin Psychiatry. 2004;65(5):611–7.
13. Butterweck V, Schmidt M. St. John's wort: role of active compounds for its mechanism of action and efficacy. Wien Med Wochenschr. 2007;157(13–14):356–61.
14. Butterweck V. Mechanism of action of St John's wort in depression : what is known? CNS Drugs. 2003;17(8):539–62.
15. Sublette, M., S. Ellis, A. Geant and J. Mann (2011). "Meta-analysis of the effects of eicosapentaenoic acid (EPA) in clinical trials in depression." *J Clin Psychiatry* **72**(12): 1577-1584.
16. Wurglics M, Schubert-Zsilavecz M. *Hypericum perforatum*: a 'modern' herbal antidepressant: pharmacokinetics of active ingredients. Clin Pharmacokinet. 2006;45(5):449–68.
17. Schulz HU et al. Investigation of pharmacokinetic data of hypericin, pseudohypericin, hyperforin and the flavonoids quercetin and isorhamnetin revealed from single and multiple oral dose studies with a hypericum extract containing tablet in healthy male volunteers. Arzneimittelforschung. 2005;55(10):561–8.
18. Biber A. Oral bioavailability of hyperforin from hypericum extracts in rats and human volunteers. Pharmacopsychiatry. 1998;31(Suppl 1):36–43.
19. Linde K, Berner M, Kriston L. St John's wort for major depression. Cochrane Database Syst Rev. 2008;4:CD000448.
20. Rahimi R, Nikfar S, Abdollahi M. Efficacy and tolerability of *Hypericum perforatum* in major depressive disorder in comparison with selective serotonin reuptake inhibitors: a meta-analysis. Prog Neuropsychopharmacol Biol Psychiatry. 2009;33(1):118–27.
21. Taylor LH, Kobak KA. An open-label trial of St. John's Wort (*Hypericum perforatum*) in obsessive-compulsive disorder. J Clin Psychiatry. 2000;61(8):575–8.
22. Kobak KA et al. St John's wort versus placebo in obsessive-compulsive disorder: results from a double-blind study. Int Clin Psychopharmacol. 2005;20(6):299–304.
23. Kobak KA et al. St. John's wort versus placebo in social phobia: results from a placebo-controlled pilot study. J Clin Psychopharmacol. 2005;25(1):51–8.
24. Volz HP et al. St John's wort extract (LI 160) in somatoform disorders: results of a placebo-controlled trial. Psychopharmacology (Berl). 2002;164(3):294–300.
25. Muller T et al. Treatment of somatoform disorders with St. John's wort: a randomized, double-blind and placebo-controlled trial. Psychosom Med. 2004;66(4):538–47.
26. Kessler RC et al. Epidemiology of anxiety disorders. Curr Top Behav Neurosci. 2010;2:21–35.
27. Tyrer P, Baldwin D. Generalised anxiety disorder. Lancet. 2006;368(9553):2156–66.
28. Newcorn JH, Weiss M, Stein MA. The complexity of ADHD: diagnosis and treatment of the adult patient with comorbidities. CNS spectr. 2007;12(8 Suppl 12):1–14.
29. Weber W et al. *Hypericum perforatum* (St John's wort) for attention-deficit/hyperactivity disorder in children and adolescents: A randomized controlled trial. JAMA. 2008;299(22):2633–41.
30. Schmidt M, Betti G, Hensel A. Saffron in phytotherapy: pharmacology and clinical uses. Wien Med Wochenschr. 2007;157(13–14):315–9.
31. Hosseinzadeh H, Noraei NB. Anxiolytic and hypnotic effect of *Crocus sativus* aqueous extract and its constituents, crocin and safranal, in mice. Phytother Res. 2009;23(6):768–74.
32. Lechtenberg M et al. Quality and functionality of saffron: quality control, species assortment and affinity of extract and isolated saffron compounds to NMDA and sigma1 (sigma-1) receptors. Planta Med. 2008;74(7):764–72.

33. Hosseinzadeh H, Sadeghnia H. Protective effect of safranal on pentylenetetrazol-induced seizures in the rat: involvement of GABAergic and opioids systems. Phytomedicine. 2007;14(4):256–62.
34. Pathan SA et al. Quantitative analysis of safranal in saffron extract and nanoparticle formulation by a validated high-performance thin-layer chromatographic method. Phytochem Anal. 2010;21(3):219–23.
35. Ghadrdoost B et al. Protective effects of saffron extract and its active constituent crocin against oxidative stress and spatial learning and memory deficits induced by chronic stress in rats. Eur J Pharmacol. 2011;667(1–3):222–9.
36. Nam KN et al. Anti-inflammatory effects of crocin and crocetin in rat brain microglial cells. Eur J Pharmacol. 2010;648(1–3):110–6.
37. Mehri S et al. Neuroprotectiveeffect of crocin on acrylamide-induced cytotoxicity in PC12 cells.Cell MolNeurobiol. 2011;32(2):227–35.
38. Akhondzadeh S et al. *Crocus sativus* L. in the treatment of mild to moderate depression: a double-blind, randomized and placebo-controlled trial. Phytother Res. 2005;19(2):148–51.
39. Moshiri E et al. *Crocus sativus* L. (petal) in the treatment of mild-to-moderate depression: a double-blind, randomized and placebo-controlled trial. Phytomedicine. 2006;13(9–10):607–11.
40. Akhondzadeh S et al. Comparison of *Crocus sativus* L. and imipramine in the treatment of mild to moderate depression: a pilot double-blind randomized trial [ISRCTN45683816]. BMC Complement Altern Med. 2004;4:12.
41. Noorbala AA et al. Hydro-alcoholic extract of *Crocus sativus* L. versus fluoxetine in the treatment of mild to moderate depression: a double-blind, randomized pilot trial. J Ethnopharmacol. 2005;97(2):281–4.
42. Akhondzadeh B et al. Comparison of petal of *Crocus sativus* L. and fluoxetine in the treatment of depressed outpatients: a pilot double-blind randomized trial. Prog Neuropsychopharmacol Biol Psychiatry. 2007;30(2):439–42.
43. Mischoulon D, Freeman MP. Omega-3 fatty acids in psychiatry. Psychiatr Clin North Am. 2013;36(1):15–23.
44. Rapaport MH et al. Inflammation as a predictive biomarker for response to omega-3 fatty acids in major depressive disorder: a proof-of-concept study. Mol Psychiatry. 2015;21(1):71–9.
45. Raison CL, Capuron L, Miller AH. Cytokines sing the blues: inflammation and the pathogenesis of depression. Trends Immunol. 2006;27(1):24–31.
46. Tassoni D et al. The role of eicosanoids in the brain. Asia Pac J Clin Nutr. 2008;17(Suppl 1):220–8.
47. Sarris J, Mischoulon D, Schweitzer I. Omega-3 for bipolar disorder: meta-analyses of use in mania and bipolar depression. J Clin Psychiatry. 2012;73(1):81–6.
48. Stoll A. Omega-3 fatty acids in mood disorders: a review of neurobiological and clinical actions.In: Rosenbaum J,Mischoulon D, editors.Natural medications for psychiatric disorders: considering the alternatives. Philadelphia: Lippincott Williams & Wilkins;2008.p. 39–67.
49. Hamazaki K et al. Effect of omega-3 fatty acid-containing phospholipids on blood catecholamine concentrations in healthy volunteers: a randomized, placebo-controlled, double-blind trial. Nutrition. 2005;21(6):705–10.
50. Appleton KM, Rogers PJ, Ness AR. Updated systematic review and meta-analysis of the effects of n-3 long-chain polyunsaturated fatty acids on depressed mood. Am J Clin Nutr. 2010;91(3):757–70.
51. Lin PY et al. Are omega-3 fatty acids antidepressants or just mood-improving agents? The effect depends upon diagnosis, supplement preparation, and severity of depression. Mol Psychiatry. 2012;17(12):1161–3 ; author reply 1163–7.
52. Sarris, J., J. Murphy, D. Mischoulon, M. Fava, M. Berk and C. Ng (2016). "Adjunctive Nutrient Nutraceuticals for Depression: A Systematic Review and Meta-analyses." *The American Journal Of Psychiatry*; 1;173(6):575-87.
53. Martins JG. EPA but not DHA appears to be responsible for the efficacy of omega-3 long chain polyunsaturated fatty acid supplementation in depression: evidence from a meta-analysis of randomized controlled trials. J Am Coll Nutr. 2009;28(5):525–42.

54. Mischoulon D et al. A double-blind, randomized controlled clinical trial comparing eicosapentaenoic acid versus docosahexaenoic acid for depression. J Clin Psychiatry. 2015;76(1):54–61.
55. Papakostas GI. Evidence for S-adenosyl-L-methionine (SAM-e) for the treatment of major depressive disorder. J Clin Psychiatry. 2009;70(Suppl 5):18–22.
56. Fava M, Mischoulon D. Folate in depression: efficacy, safety, differences in formulations, and clinical issues. J Clin Psychiatry. 2009;70(Suppl 5):12–7.
57. Alpert JE et al. Folinic acid (Leucovorin) as an adjunctive treatment for SSRI-refractory depression. Ann Clin Psychiatry. 2002;14(1):33–8.
58. Papakostas GI et al. L-methylfolate as adjunctive therapy for SSRI-resistant major depression: results of two randomized, double-blind, parallel-sequential trials. Am J Psychiatry. 2012;169(12):1267–74.
59. Williams AL et al. S-adenosylmethionine (SAMe) as treatment for depression: a systematic review. Clin Invest Med. 2005;28(3):132–9.
60. Baek J, Bernstein E, Nierenberg A. One-carbon metabolism and bipolar disorder. Aust N Z J Psychiatry. 2013;47(11):1013–8.
61. Genedani S et al. Influence of SAMe on the modifications of brain polyamine levels in an animal model of depression. Neuroreport. 2001;12(18):3939–42.
62. Zomkowski AD, Santos AR, Rodrigues AL. Putrescine produces antidepressant-like effects in the forced swimming test and in the tail suspension test in mice. Prog Neuropsychopharmacol Biol Psychiatry. 2006;30(8):1419–25.
63. Berlanga C et al. Efficacy of S-adenosyl-L-methionine in speeding the onset of action of imipramine. Psychiatry Res. 1992;44(3):257–62.
64. Papakostas GI et al. S-adenosyl methionine (SAMe) augmentation of serotonin reuptake inhibitors for antidepressant nonresponders with major depressive disorder: a double-blind, randomized clinical trial. Am J Psychiatry. 2010;167(8):942–8.
65. Mischoulon D et al. A Double-blind, randomized, placebo-controlled clinical trial of S-adenosyl-L-methionine (SAMe) versus escitalopram in major depressive disorder. J Clin Psychiatry2014;75(4):370–6.
66. Sarris J et al. S-adenosyl methionine (SAMe) versus escitalopram and placebo in major depression: efficacy and effects of histamine and carnitine as moderators of response. J Affect Disord. 2014;164:76–81.
67. Sarris J, Price LH, Carpenter L, Tyrka AR, Ng CH, Papakostas GI, Jaeger A, Fava M, Mischoulon D. Is S-adenosyl methionine (SAMe) for depression only effective in males? A re-analysis of data from a randomized clinical trial. Pharmacopsychiatry. 2015;48(4–5):141–4.
68. Mischoulon D, Raab MF. The role of folate in depression and dementia. J Clin Psychiatry. 2007;68(Suppl 10):28–33.
69. Deligiannidis KM, Freeman MP. Complementary and alternative medicine for the treatment of depressive disorders in women. Psychiatr Clin North Am. 33(2):441–63.
70. Spillmann M, Fava M. S-adenosyl-methionine (ademethionine) in psychiatric disorders. CNS Drugs. 1996;6:416–25.
71. Carrieri P et al. S-adenosylmethionine treatment of depressioin in patients with Parkinson's disease: a double-blind, crossover study versus placebo. Curr Ther Res. 1990;48(1):154–60.
72. Di Rocco A et al. Adenosyl-Methionine improves depression in patients with Parkinson's disease in an open-label clinical trial. Mov Disord. 2000;15(6):1225–9.
73. Szewczyk B, Kubera M, Nowak G. The role of zinc in neurodegenerative inflammatory pathways in depression. Prog Neuropsychopharmacol Biol Psychiatry. 2011;35(3):693–701.
74. Swardfager W et al. Potential roles of zinc in the pathophysiology and treatment of major depressive disorder. Neurosci Biobehav Rev. 2013;37(5):911–29.
75. Prasad AS. Zinc: role in immunity, oxidative stress and chronic inflammation. Curr Opin Clin Nutr Metab Care. 2009;12(6):646–52.

76. Yary T, Aazami S. Dietary intake of zinc was inversely associated with depression. Biol Trace Elem Res. 2011;145(3):286–90.
77. Swardfager W et al. Zinc in depression: a meta-analysis. Biol Psychiatry. 2013;74(12):872–8.
78. Lai J et al. The efficacy of zinc supplementation in depression: systematic review of randomised controlled trials. J Affect Disord. 2012;136(1–2):e31–9.
79. Cunha MP et al. Interaction of zinc with antidepressants in the tail suspension test. Prog Neuropsychopharmacol Biol Psychiatry. 2008;32(8):1913–20.
80. Barrie SA et al. Comparative absorption of zinc picolinate, zinc citrate and zinc gluconate in humans. Agents Actions. 1987;21(1–2):223–8.
81. Mischoulon D, Fava M. Role of S-adenosyl-L-methionine in the treatment of depression: a review of the evidence. Am J Clin Nutr. 2002;76(5):1158S–61S.
82. Sarris J. Current challenges in appraising complementary medicine evidence. MJA. 2012;196(5):310–1.
83. Izzo AA. Drug interactions with St. John's Wort (*Hypericum perforatum*): a review of the clinical evidence. Int J Clin Pharmacol Ther. 2004;42(3):139–48.
84. Whitten D et al. The effect of St John's wort extracts on CYP3A: a systematic review of prospective clinical trials. Br J Clin Pharmacol. 2006;62(5):512–26.
85. FDA. http://www.fda.gov/Food/FoodIngredientsPackaging/GenerallyRecognizedasSafeGRAS/default.htm. 2012.
86. Modaghegh MH et al. Safety evaluation of saffron (*Crocus sativus*) tablets in healthy volunteers. Phytomedicine. 2008;15(12):1032–7.

Part II

Traditional Treatments in Need of Further Study

The Therapeutic Potential of Ayahuasca

7

Michael A. Coe and Dennis J. McKenna

7.1 Introduction

Ayahuasca is a Quechua term that is commonly translated into "vine of the spirits, vine of the soul, or vine of the dead" and refers to jungle liana in the Malpighiaceae family taxonomically known as *Banisteriopsiscaapi* Spruce ex. Griseb. The same term is synonymous with a psychoactive tea or beverage traditionally used by cultural groups throughout parts of Brazil, Peru, Colombia, Bolivia, Venezuela, and Ecuador during rites of passage, divination, warfare, magico-religious practices, and for healing in the context of ethnomedical practices [1–4]. Traditional preparations of *ayahuasca* tea include the combination of bark and stems of the *Banisteriopsis caapi* liana plus admixture plants; most commonly the leaves of *Psychotria viridis* Ruiz & Pav. (Rubiaceae) or *Diplopterys cabrerana* (Cuatrec.) B. Gates (Malpighiaceae) are boiled and reduced for several hours [5].

7.1.1 Constituents

Bioactive investigations of *ayahuasca* have revealed a unique synergistic chemistry and pharmacology in regard to its source and admixture plants. The leaves of *P. viridis* and *D. cabrerana* contain a highly potent, typically short-acting

M.A. Coe, PhD (✉)
Department of Botany, University of Hawai`i at Mānoa,
3190 Maile Way, St. John, Room 101, 96822 Honolulu, HI, USA
e-mail: coem@hawaii.edu

D.J. McKenna, PhD
Center for Spirituality & Healing, University of Minnesota, Academic Health Center,
Mayo Mail Code 505, 420 Delaware St., Minneapolis, MN 55455, USA
e-mail: mcken031@umn.edu

D. Camfield et al. (eds.), *Evidence-Based Herbal and Nutritional Treatments for Anxiety in Psychiatric Disorders*, DOI 10.1007/978-3-319-42307-4_7

psychoactive alkaloid N, N-dimethyltryptamine (DMT) [6]. Research suggests, when ingested orally DMT is rendered inactive by monoamine oxidase (MAO) in the gut and liver [5]. However, when combined with the monoamine oxidase inhibitor (MAOI) beta-carbolines (harmine, harmaline, and tetrahydroharmine) present within the bark and stems of *B. caapi*, DMT is protected from peripheral degradation and becomes orally active, crossing the blood–brain barrier intact via active transport [5–7].

It is important to mention that cultural groups may utilize different concentrations of source plants as well as employ various admixture plants in preparation of *ayahuasca*, which may affect its overall pharmacological activity [5, 8]. Additionally, these cultural groups may exhibit a range of ethnotaxonomy in regard to the vine as well as the tea, making the distinction between the two rather complex [3]. For example, the vernacular terms *hoasca, caapi, natéma, pildé, daime*, and *vegetal* refer to the tea whereas *ayahuasca*, *yage, cielo, trueno, negra, boa, tigrehuasca, culbrahuasca*, and *intihuasca* are synonymous with both the tea and the Banisteriopsis liana [3, 4, 9–11].

7.1.2 Mechanisms of Action

In regard to the putative mechanisms of action by which *ayahuasca* may influence mood and anxiety, the beta-carbolines (primarily harmine, harmaline, and tetrahydroharmine) have the potential to facilitate an increased density of 5-HT transporters in the prefrontal cortex, while additionally acting as serotonin reuptake and MAO inhibitors [4, 5, 12]. Specifically, the beta-carbolines present in *ayahuasca* have been shown to be reversible competitive peripheral MAO-A inhibitors that may enhance levels of endogenous serotonin and catecholamines [4, 12, 13], whereas DMT present in *ayahuasca* is structurally related to serotonin and has been shown to induce bioactive responses in the central nervous system where it interacts with 5-$HT_{2A/1A/2C}$ receptor sites [12–14]. It has been suggested that the inhibition of serotonin reuptake and MAO induced by *ayahuasca* may result in increased levels of brain serotonin [4, 15]. In addition, preclinical evidence suggests that harmine may play a significant role in the treatment of depression. Preliminary studies suggest that harmine has an affinity for Imidazoline (I2) binding sites that are considered integral target sites for antidepressants [16]. In animal models it has been noted that harmine may increase hippocampal brain-derived neurotrophic factor (BDNF) levels, superoxidase dismutase, and catalase activity, which are thought to contribute to its antidepressant effects [16].

7.2 Psycho-Socio-Cultural Significance of Ayahuasca and Scheduling of DMT

In order to understand the psycho-socio-cultural significance of *ayahuasca* as well as its therapeutic potential among cultural groups and practitioners that utilize it, it is important to consider the lenses from which it is viewed; in particular, both the emic (perception from the eyes of a cultural group) and etic (perception from the eyes of an outside observer) perspectives. The emic perspective suggests that *ayahuasca* is considered the cosmo-vision of the Amazonian people, an entity or spiritual being, a powerful plant teacher, a religious sacrament, and a medicine [5, 8, 10, 17, 18]. The etic perspective of *ayahuasca* is one that is dualistic in nature as it has long been a focus of scientific inquiry since its discovery due to its reported uses as a great medicine to diagnose and treat illness [1, 11, 19].

In contrast, there has been notable controversy regarding the legal status of *ayahuasca*. Although *ayahuasca* and its source plants are not internationally prohibited under the 1971 International Convention on Psychotropic Substances, one of the principal ingredients *P. viridis* or the alternative DMT-admixture plant used in some regions *D. cabrerana* contains the psychoactive alkaloid DMT [6]. Extracted DMT has been classified by regulatory agencies in the United States as a Schedule 1 controlled substance and is listed as a controlled substance under the International Convention on Psychotropic Substances [5]. The scheduling of DMT, which has defined it as a "drug and substance of abuse," has undoubtedly influenced the public perception of *ayahuasca* as these terms may carry cultural connotations. Furthermore, it has been suggested that the classification of DMT as a drug and substance of abuse is based on sociopolitical agendas rather that scientific evidence [see 7 for suggested literature]. Although the legal definition of the term "drug" includes organic substances used to treat illness, it is highly probable that anyone who has been exposed to the "War on Drugs," an antidrug campaign made popular by the U.S. Nixon Administration in 1971, have been predisposed to cultural programming in regard to these terms.

It is noteworthy to mention that botanical sources of DMT and moreover *ayahuasca* have not been listed as controlled substances nor regulated as such by international regulatory agencies [5]. Interestingly, research has shown that DMT is not only found in plants but is also present in mammals, amphibians, and occurs endogenous within humans and other animals, including the blood, brain, lungs, adrenals, and cerebrospinal fluid [4]. Additionally, botanical sources of DMT have been shown to be nontoxic within the human system and there is no evidence to indicate that DMT is addictive, either psychologically or physiologically [7]. Endogenous DMT found within the human system may also play a role in cell protection, immune response, and regeneration due to its affinity for Sig-1R receptors at the endoplasmic reticulum–mitochondria interface [7].

In light of these findings, it is reasonable to propose that studies regarding the functional role DMT plays within the human system as well as *ayahuasca* have an important contribution in the fields of ethnopharmacology, neuroscience, and psychiatry. Nevertheless, scheduling of DMT as well as the cultural lenses, which perceive it solely for its psychoactive effects, have superficially made human biochemistry illegal to study and have led to few rigorous scientific studies conducted on the therapeutic potential of *ayahuasca* as well as the biodynamic role DMT may play within the human system. The following section is a brief overview of the current therapeutic applications of *ayahuasca* to treat addiction, depression, and anxiety. In this context, the authors highlight studies that help to facilitate a greater understanding of the therapeutic potential of *ayahuasca*, while also encouraging an open dialogue relating to its potential applications in medical practice.

7.3 Modern Uses of Ayahuasca

After the European involvement associated with the rubber booms in the Amazon (1879–1912 and 1945–1947), several prominent syncretic religious movements formed in Brazil during the twentieth century began to use *ayahuasca* independently from the traditional indigenous practices [20]. The *União de Vegetal* (UDV), the *Santo Daime*, and the *Barquinha* utilize *ayahuasca* as a sacrament within a healing and religious context. These churches incorporate a complex integration of Afro-Brazilian cosmologies, Catholic and European esoteric traditions, and indigenous knowledge of plant use within their religious practices [4, 20, 21]. Among these groups, *ayahuasca* is consumed on a regular basis and is symbolically equivalent to that of the Christian Eucharist [1, 5]. Although the *Barquinha* have remained a more localized religious organization in Brazil, the *Santo Daime* and UDV have become established in more than 23 countries including Japan, Germany, South Africa, Spain, Canada, and Holland [16, 22]. In addition, both the *Santo Daime* and the UDV have more recently become active religious organizations in the United States under the Religious Freedom Restoration Act of 1993 [5]. It is important to mention that the consumption of *ayahuasca* among church members has been reported to have no known deleterious effects. Further, it has been reported that members of the UDV that have consumed *ayahuasca* regularly for decades show signs of physical vigor and mental acuity, and also a low incidence of serious *illness* [5, 6].

The centuries of European acculturation of the Amazon have led to the development of a Mestizo ethnomedical tradition known as *vegetalismo*. *Vegetalismo* is a ritualistic healing tradition that is over 100 years old, and comprises traditional indigenous Amazonian use of *ayahuasca* and admixture plants, together with Christian beliefs, and Andean influences [3, 17]. The use of *ayahuasca* among practitioners of *vegetalismo*, plant specialists known as *vegetalistas*, is akin to that of the traditional cultural use. In many communities in the Amazon region that have limited access to Western medicine, the *vegetalista* assumes the role of healer, psychotherapist, and spiritual guide [2]. In this context, *ayahuasca* and admixture plants are used for the diagnosis and treatment of illness, divination, and a gateway to supernatural realms [3, 5, 17, 23, 24]. In terms of the use of *ayahuasca* aimed toward diagnosis and the treatment of illness, *vegetalistas* have adopted a holistic approach similar to that of the naturopathic trend in modern medicine in that it recognizes a mind/body interconnection that is intrinsically tied to concepts of illness. To the *vegetalistas*, illness may stem from physiological, psychological, and or supernatural causes.

It is important to mention that *vegetalistas* utilize *ayahuasca* primarily to determine sources of illness within their patients; after which they may employ a variety of methods for treatment including the use of medicinal plants, magical chants, and/-or incantations [17]. The most comprehensive study to date suggests that *vegetalistas* incorporate a vast ethnopharmacopeia comprising of over 50 genera of plants within their ethnomedical practices [2]. Although the use of *ayahuasca* within the *vegetalismo* tradition has been well-documented, few rigorous studies have been conducted to investigate the use of admixture plants within Mestizo ethnomedicine. Additional research is warranted to determine the chemistry and pharmacology of admixture plants as well as their efficacy and potential therapeutic uses.

The use of *ayahuasca* has entered into the global sphere with the expansion of the religious sects mentioned above, as well as the rise of a phenomenon known as "*ayahuasca tourism*." In regard to *ayahuasca* tourism, it is quite common for people from other countries and differing socioeconomic backgrounds to travel to the Peruvian Amazon to drink *ayahuasca* [3]. Ethnographic studies suggest that in this context *ayahuasca* is consumed in a ritualistic setting, often guided by Mestizo or indigenous *ayahuasqueros* (one who uses *ayahuasca* in a ritualistic healing context), and is used to facilitate self-transformation, physical, psychological, and spiritual healing, as well as an increased sense of well-being among participants [11, 24]. Contrary to the belief that participants who attend *ayahuasca* retreats are motivated to utilize *ayahuasca* for recreational purposes associated with the concept of "drug tourism," research has demonstrated that the majority of participants are motivated by intentions to seek increased self-awareness, insights that may enhance personal growth, and a spiritual connection with the natural world [25]. Interestingly, there have been reports of participants purging physical, psychological, and emotional imbalances [11, 24]. However, further research is needed in order to evaluate both the physiological and psychological implications of the ritualistic therapeutic use of *ayahuasca* associated with *ayahuasca* tourism.

7.4 Evidence of Efficacy

Despite an increased global interest regarding the therapeutic potential of *ayahuasca*, few rigorous modern scientific studies have been conducted in order to evaluate its efficacy to treat physiological and or psychological disorders defined under Western classification systems (i.e, DSM or ICD). However, over the last 20 years, preliminary investigations have been conducted including the following: (1) clinical trials investigating the potential deleterious and therapeutic effects of *ayahuasca* among active members of both the UDV and *Santo Daime*, (2) treatment protocols assessing the therapeutic potential of the ritualistic *ayahuasca* use in addressing drug and alcohol addiction, and (3) pharmacological investigations that aim to elucidate the biodynamic mechanisms of *ayahuasca* within the human system as well as their potential to play a role in the treatment of addiction, depression, and anxiety.

7.4.1 Therapeutic Effects Observed in the "*Hoasca* Project"

Beginning in the late 1990s, researchers adopted a multidisciplinary approach to evaluate the short- and long-term toxicology profiles of active members of the Brazilian UDV, who had regularly ingested *ayahuasca* for 10 or more years [1, 5].

The "*Hoasca* Project" was comprised of physiological and neuropsychological assessments, personality testing, and psychiatric evaluations of 15 long-term UDV church members who consumed *ayahuasca* (or *hoasca* as it is known in Brazil) as a religious sacrament. These assessments were compared to 15 control subjects that did not use *Hoasca* but were matched according to age and socioeconomic status [1, 4, 5, 21]. Grob et al. [1] found no data to suggest there was either short- or long-term toxicity among participants in the study. Additionally, there was no evidence of deleterious health effects [1, 5]. Perhaps the most promising findings of the *Hoasca* Project were the implications of a therapeutic potential. Prior to induction into the religion and long-term use of *hoasca*, a majority of members reported previous histories of alcoholism and tobacco addiction [1]. In addition, several members mentioned during life history interviews either a prior diagnosis of a drug addiction, an anxiety disorder, a history of domestic violence, or a significant depressive disorder [1, 4, 5, 21]. These dysfunctional lifestyle behaviors and psychiatric disorders were reported to have ceased following the regular use of *ayahuasca* within a religious context [1].

While it is feasible to suggest that the positive lifestyle changes exhibited by the church members in this study may be due in part to other factors such as the social support associated with church affiliation, measurements of serotonergic function within the members of the study suggested direct psychopharmacological effects. Previous research has shown that deficits and genetic polymorphisms in the 5-HT serotonin reuptake transporters are associated with the aggressive and violent behaviors exhibited by type II alcoholics and individuals with substance dependence as well as heightened states of anxiety [4, 5, 26–28]. In addition, low abundance of serotonin transporters as well as disrupted serotonergic neurotransmission have been shown to correlate with impulsive and severe antisocial behaviors, acute depression, suicidal tendencies, as well as homicidal behaviors [15, 27, 28]. It has been suggested that a long-term effect of ingesting certain phytochemical constituents of *ayahuasca* (e.g., MAOI's and/or DMT) may play a role in serotonin transporter gene expression and contribute to the favorable lifestyle changes such as those observed among UDV church members [4, 5, 29].

Callaway et al. [29] reported that regular consumption of *ayahuasca* by participants involved in the *Hoasca project* was associated with an increase in serotonin reuptake transporters within blood platelets. This finding pertained to members of the UDV who had consumed *hoasca* for 10 years or more compared to age-matched *ayahuasca*-naïve subjects [15, 29]. While this study did not provide a direct measure of serotonin reuptake transporters within the central nervous system and brain, it is noteworthy that increased serotonin reuptake transporters in blood platelets are correlated with transporters in the brain [15]. This suggests that the regular consumption of *ayahuasca* may have the potential to reverse deficits in serotonergic neurotransmission. To date, *ayahuasca* is perhaps the only natural botanically derived substance known to upregulate serotonin transporters and may prove to be one of the mechanisms that contribute to its putative therapeutic properties [5, 15].

7.4.2 Anxiety and Panic

In a study of members of the *Santo Daime*, Santos et al. [4] also investigated the potential therapeutic effects associated with long-term *ayahuasca* use. The emotional states that were investigated included anxiety, panic, and depression, the symptoms of which were typically diminished with treatment by serotonin agonists and reuptake inhibitors [see 4 for suggested literature]. In consideration of the proposed mechanisms by which the phytochemical constituents of *ayahuasca* interact with human physiology and facilitate serotonergic transmission, it is feasible to suggest that the regular long-term use of *ayahuasca* may attenuate the symptoms pertaining to the emotional states linked to anxiety, panic, and depression [4, 5]. Using a rigorous double-blind, placebo-controlled design, Santos et al. [4] utilized psychometric measures to evaluate anxiety, panic states, and depression among nine psychologically healthy long-term members of the *Santo Daime* that regularly ingested *ayahuasca* as a religious sacrament for over 10 years. This study was conducted over a 3-week period during which psychometric subscales were employed including the state–trait–anxiety inventory (STAI) to measure state/trait-anxiety, the anxiety sensitivity index (ASI) to measure panic-like states correlated with anxiety sensitivity and panic disorder, and the Beck hopeless scale (BHS) to measure symptoms associated with hopelessness (i.e., clinical depression). All participants were administered treatments consisting of either a placebo/inactive solution, a full-*ayahuasca* solution, or an *ayahuasca*-flavored solution. It is important to mention that each treatment was administered to participants in a crossover placebo-controlled study design with a week between each dose. Results indicated a significant reduction in panic-like states and hopelessness (depression) was observed for *Santo Daime* members in comparison to controls [4], although little evidence was found to support diminished state or trait anxiety. However, the authors note that these results may be attributed to long-term users of *ayahuasca* exhibiting low levels of anxiety traits at baseline [4].

A more recent study conducted by Fernández et al. [30] suggests that diminished states of anxiety were associated with *ayahuasca* use, according to psychopathology subscales used to assess the ritualistic use of *ayahuasca* for treatment of substance dependence. The psychopathological status, personality traits, neuropsychological performance and behavior, as well as the life attitudes and psychosocial well-being of each participant were assessed via the *Symptom Check-List-90-Revised* (SCL-90-R), *Temperament and Character Inventory* (TCI-Revised), *Stroop Color and Word Test*, and the *Purpose in Life Test* (PLT), respectively. Data collection for this study was performed for approximately 4 years and participants ingested *ayahuasca* treatments approximately 2–3 times per month on average. In addition, a recent study by Osório et al. [31], which investigated the antidepressant effects of a single-dose treatment of *ayahuasca*, demonstrated a significant reduction in anxiety and depression symptoms as assessed using the Brief Psychiatric Rating Scale (BPRS).

7.4.3 Depression

A preliminary study on the therapeutic potential of *ayahuasca* for the treatment of depression was recently conducted on three female participants diagnosed with mild-to-severe depressive disorders. De Lima Osório et al. [32] utilized the Hamilton-D psychiatric rating scale (HAM-D) to evaluate participants 10 min prior to receiving a single dose of 2 ml/kg of *ayahuasca*; after which participants were evaluated 40, 80, 140, and 180 min after ingestion. Follow-up evaluations of the participants using (HAM-D) were conducted 1, 2, 4, 7, 14, and 28 days after the initial treatment. A significant decrease in HAM-D scores was observed, an effect that lasted up to 14 days following the consumption of *ayahuasca* [32].

As mentioned previously, Osório et al. [31] investigated the therapeutic potential of *ayahuasca* in the treatment of depression using six participants previously diagnosed with a recurrent mild depressive disorder. Participants were administered a single dose of *ayahuasca* 2.2 ml/kg and assessed using psychiatric measures including (BPRS), Young Mania Rating Scale (YMRS), (HAM-D), and the Montgomery-Asberg Depression Rating Scale (MADRS). Assessments were taken at 10 min prior to ingestion (baseline), as well as at 40, 80, 140, and 180 min post-dose. Follow-up assessments were also conducted 1, 7, 14, and 21 day(s) following treatment using the same outcome measures. It is noteworthy that prior to treatment with *ayahuasca*, two participants reported a mild depressive episode, three reported a moderate depressive episode, and one reported a severe depressive episode [31].

Osório et al. [31] have reported significant reductions in depressive symptoms (82 %) according to (HAM-D), (MADRS), and BPRS Anxious-Depression subscale. These reductions were observed between baseline and 1, 7, and 21 day(s) following treatment with *ayahuasca*. Critically, no significant changes to YMRS (i.e., elevated mood, increased activity and energy, sexual interest, sleep, irritability, speech, language-thought disorder, thought contents, aggressive and disruptive behavior, appearance, and insight) were observed, suggesting that *ayahuasca* does not induce mania/hypomania in patients previously diagnosed with a mood disorder. Additionally, there were also nonsignificant changes according to thinking disorder measures assessed by the (BPRS), which the authors speculated may indicate that thought content modifications induced by psychoactive effects were not critical for mood improvement [31]. This finding of significant reductions in anxiety and depression symptoms between 140 min and 7 days following treatment with *ayahuasca* suggests that the acute antidepressant and anxiolytic effects of *ayahuasca* occur rapidly compared to clinically prescribed antidepressants [31]. For example, the most common prescribed medications for the treatment of depressive disorder include selective serotonin reuptake inhibitors (SSRIs) such as fluoxetine and citalopram that have been shown to increase levels of serotonin in the short-term however, may take up to 2 weeks on average for the onset of therapeutic action and in the long-term are likely to downregulate serotonin transporters [31, 33]. Finally, although the sample size in the studies mentioned above was limited, future research utilizing larger sample size as well as a double-blind, placebo-controlled protocol is warranted.

7.4.4 Substance Dependence

Perhaps one of the more promising therapeutic applications of *ayahuasca* may be for the treatment of addiction. Several *ayahuasca* treatment centers, most notably the *Takiwasi* (Quechua term meaning "house that sings") Center for Drug Addict Rehabilitation located in Peru, have adopted an integrated approach toward treating addiction through the ritualistic use of *ayahuasca* [8, 34, 35]. Founded in 1992 and led by Dr. Jacques Mabit, the Takiwasi center has specialized in the treatment of substance and alcohol dependence for over 20 years [8, 21, 35]. An integral and novel component of the *Takiwasi* program is the integration of the ritualistic use of *ayahuasca* and other plants as guided by a traditional healer, together with a treatment model consisting of psychotherapy and elements of social cohesion, factors which have been attributed to its success [see 34, 35 for a detailed description of program protocol]. Although the center has yet to conduct formal clinical trials and produce peer-reviewed data, the program reports encouraging evidence of initial clinical success. It has been noted that within 5 years of the *Takiwasi* programs inception, 67 % of the 175 patients exhibiting substance and or alcohol dependence have avoided relapse after 2 years of completing treatment protocols [16].

Adopting an interdisciplinary approach similar to the *Takiwasi* Program, an initial observational study of *ayahuasca*-based treatments for substance dependence was conducted on members of the First Nations community in British Columbia, Canada [36]. This study consisted of methodologies involving the ritualistic use of *ayahuasca* during two sessions guided by a traditional healer along with psychological and behavioral assessments on 12 *ayahuasca*-naïve subjects that demonstrated problematic substance abuse. Pretreatment and 6-month follow-up data resulted in significant improvements in a range of psychological outcome measures [36]. Participants in the program demonstrated increased scores on psychotherapeutic measurement scales, which assessed empowerment, mindfulness, hopefulness, quality of life meaning, and outlook. Additionally, participants self-reported a significant reduction in cocaine, tobacco, and alcohol use whereas the use of opiates and cannabis did not diminish. It is important to note that the authors mention that the continued use of cannabis and opiates were in some cases due to medical prescription [36]. These preliminary findings are promising, although further research using an age-matched control group is warranted.

Another preliminary study conducted by Fernández et al. [30] at the Institute for Applied Amazonian Ethnopsychology (IDEAA) utilized personality, psychopathology, and neuropsychological measurements to assess the effects of the ritualistic use of *ayahuasca* on substance dependence. Thirteen participants were administered biweekly *ayahuasca*-based treatments at both the IDEEA and a *Santo Daime* community that lasting 3 and 9 months. Of the 13 participants, nine were diagnosed with problematic substance dependence (heroin/cocaine derivatives) and one with borderline personality disorder (BPD). The remaining three participants received *ayahuasca*-based treatments for personal development [30]. Personality, psychopathology, and neuropsychological measures were assessed using the following scales/subscales: Temperament and Character-Inventory Revised (TCI-R),

Symptom-Checklist- 90-Revised (SCL-90R), Stroop Color and Word Test, Letter Number Sequencing (LNS) from the WAIS-III, Frontal Systems Behavioral Scale (FrSBe), Purpose in Life Test (PLT), and Spiritual Orientation Inventory (SOI) [30]. All data were analyzed using student's T test prior to and following *ayahuasca*-based treatments. Results of personality assessments revealed a significant reduction in "*Anticipatory Worry*," "*Shyness with Strangers*," and "*Disorderliness*." Similarly, psychopathological assessments showed significant symptom reductions in "*Positive Systems Total*," "*Obsessive Compulsive*," and "*Anxiety*." Additional assessments of neuropsychological performance and behavior demonstrated a significant increase in "*Resistance to Interference*" as well as significant decreases in "*Apathy*," "*Executive Dysfunction*" and "*Disinhibition*." According to the subscales used to measure life attitudes and spirituality, the data revealed a significant increase in "*Mission in Life*," "*Meaning and Purpose in Life*," "*Sacredness in Life*," "*Transcendent Dimension*," and "*Fruits of Spirituality*" [30]. Results from this study demonstrate that *ayahuasca* can contribute to significant positive behavioral improvements in psychological factors linked to substance dependence [30]. Additionally, participants exhibited less anxiety states and shyness following *ayahuasca*-based treatments. Although there were several notable limitations to this study including a limited sample size and the absence of a control group, results from this preliminary study demonstrate that the ritualistic use of *ayahuasca* in a therapeutic context may have positive behavioral and psychotherapeutic effects.

One of the most comprehensive studies to date regarding the efficacy for *ayahuasca* to treat substance dependence was conducted on church members of the CEFLURIS, a denomination of the *Santo Daime* [37]. Researchers utilized the Diagnostic and Statistical Manual for Mental Disorders (DSM-IV) to assess prior and current substance dependence among 83 participants at the moment of their induction into the religious sect. Forty-four percent of the participants were active church members for 3 years. An initial assessment was conducted to evaluate the number of participants that met the criteria for prior substance dependence. Additionally, assessments were conducted to evaluate remission criteria (i.e., a particular substance of abuse no longer being used by an individual). Out of 41 participants that met criteria for prior substance dependence, 90 % were reported to have ceased substance abuse, while 10 % were reported to exhibit continued substance abuse [37]. Subsequent data analyses revealed 27 % of the participants that met criteria for prior substance dependence were reported to have discontinued alcohol abuse, 19 % reported to have ceased habitual tobacco use, 21 % recovered from cocaine dependence, 8 % recovered from crack cocaine dependence, and 5 % recovered from dependence to other substances including heroin, LSD, solvents, and MDMA [see 8, 37 for a detailed discussion]. Although results from the studies mentioned above suggest the efficacy of *ayahuasca*-based treatments for substance dependence, it is important for future studies to consider the social aspects of community involvement and the potential synergistic effects of both the ritualistic use of *ayahuasca* and social parameters in treatment protocols. Given the implications of these preliminary reports future research is needed to assess the therapeutic efficacy of the use of *ayahuasca* within this context.

A growing interest in *ayahuasca*-based treatments for substance dependence has prompted further investigation of the potential neuropharmacological activity induced by *ayahuasca*. As a result, there have been several proposed hypotheses regarding the mechanisms for *ayahuasca* to treat substance dependence [22]. Although, clinical evidence suggests that 5-HT2A receptor-mediated antagonist may play a role as pharmacotherapeutics for the treatment for substance dependence, a recent review of clinical trials by Brierley and Davidson [16] suggests 5-HT2A agonists may prove to have greater efficacy. In addition, Liester and Prickett [22] have noted multiple neuropharmacological mechanisms by which the known agonists for 5-HT2A serotonergic receptor sites present within *ayahuasca* (e.g., DMT) may play a fundamental role in the reduction of dopamine levels in the mesolimbic brain pathway or (MBP). Previous research supports this theoretical framework in that the use of *ayahuasca* has been found to result in increased levels of prolactin, which are linked to decreased levels of dopamine in the MBP [8, 22, 38]. As a result of the proposed neuropharmacological activity of *ayahuasca*, it has been suggested that the decreased dopamine levels in the MBP would reduce the reward and or pleasure stimuli associated with substance abuse [22]. Additionally, Liester and Prickett [22] propose that the reduction of dopamine levels in the MBP may result in interference with synaptic activity directly correlated to the development and maintenance of substance dependence. Further, the authors propose that *ayahuasca* may contribute to adaptive neuroplastic changes within the dopaminergic system and facilitate the formation of new neural networks, which may result in an increase of positive adaptive behavioral responses and decrease in dysfunctional behaviors associated with substance dependence [see 22, 35 for further details]. Future research is needed to test these proposed neuropharmacological frameworks and to further assess the potential therapeutic applications of *ayahuasca*.

7.5 Conclusion and Clinical Considerations

The therapeutic potential and widespread use of *ayahuasca* has led to the development of a new cultural paradigm; one by which traditional ethnomedical knowledge and the sophisticated use of sacred medicinal plants have coevolved with multidisciplinary approaches of integrated medical practices. Given the results from the studies mentioned above there is no doubt that *ayahuasca* may prove to be an effective quintessential component in the fields of ethnopharmacology, biomedicine, and psychiatry. Although the results from preliminary investigations show great promise and suggest the efficacy of therapeutic applications of *ayahuasca* to treat substance dependence, depression, and anxiety (Table 7.1), further rigorous studies are needed to test these implications.

In light of the widespread use of *ayahuasca* in a context of a changing world, there are important clinical considerations in terms of the potential adverse effects of *ayahuasca* use in combination with antidepressants, hypnotics and sedatives, and/or alcohol. It has been cautioned that the use of ayahuasca in conjunction with SSRI type antidepressants may result in "*serotonin syndrome*"due to the

Table 7.1 Data on the therapeutic potential of ayahuasca

Herbal medicine	Dosage	Major/Active Constituents	Key evidence	Potential AEs	Potential clinical use	Clinical advice
Ayahuasca (*Psychotria viridis* plus *Banisteriopsis caapi*; or *B. caapi* plus *Diplopterys cabrerana*)	Variable dosage	MAOI: Harmine, harmaline, and tetrahydroharmine Dimethyltryptamine (DMT)	Upregulation of serotonin transporters; Research indicates anxiolytic effects and therapeutic potential to treat depression as well as substance dependence	Adverse reactions associated with "*serotonin syndrome*" have been reported when used in conjunction with SSRIs	Panic Disorder, Hoplessness, Treatment for substance dependence (cocaine, crack cocaine, alcohol, tobacco)	Important to consider *set* and *setting*. May have adverse effects if use is in close proximity to that of SSRIs, alcohol, hypnotics and sedatives. Future clinical research is warranted

mechanistic action of both DMT as a 5-HT agonists and the inhibition of metabolic breakdown of serotonin transporters by MAOI [15, 39]. Further, it has been noted that the potential adverse effects from active metabolites may persist up to 5 weeks after discontinued use of SSRIs [39]; therefore, individuals employing the use of *ayahuasca* as a complementary approach to conventional psychotherapy and/or personal development should take the necessary precautions. In addition, in order to maximize harm reduction it is important for *ayahuasca* users to consider other potentially adverse interactions with the combination of *ayahuasca* and other drugs such as alcohol and certain foods. This said, there is perhaps wisdom in traditional dietary proscriptions employed by cultural practitioners (i.e., *vegetalistas*) who have long been aware of the potential adverse effects of the combination of *ayahuasca* and these substances – an area also in need of further investigation.

References

1. Grob CS et al. Human psychopharmacology of hoasca, a plant hallucinogen used in ritual context in Brazil. J Nerv Ment Dis. 1996;184(2):86–94.
2. McKenna DJ, Luna LE, Towers GH. Biodynamic constituents in ayahuasca admixture plants. In: von Reis S, Schultes RE, editors. Ethnobotany: evolution of a discipline. Portland: Dioscorides Press; 1995.
3. Luna LE. Indigenous and mestizo use of ayahuasca: an overview. In: Santos RE d, editor. The ethnopharmacology of ayahuasca. Trivandrum: Transworld Research Network, Kerala; 2011. p. 1–21.
4. Santos RG et al. Effects of ayahuasca on psychometric measures of anxiety, panic-like and hopelessness in Santo Daime members. J Ethnopharmacol. 2007;112(3):507–13.
5. McKenna DJ. Clinical investigations of the therapeutic potential of ayahuasca: rationale and regulatory challenge. PharmacolTher. 2004;102(2):111–29.
6. Callaway JC et al. Pharmacokinetics of Hoasca alkaloids in healthy humans. J Ethnopharmacol. 1999;65(3):243–56.
7. Frecska E et al. A possibly sigma-1 receptor mediated role of dimethyltryptamine in tissue protection, regeneration, and immunity. J Neural Trans. 2013;120(9):1295–303.
8. Bouso JC, Riba J. Ayahuasca and the treatment of drug addiction. In: The therapeutic use of ayahuasca. Berlin/Heidelberg: Springer-Verlag; 2014. p. 95–109.
9. Anderson BT, Labate BC, DeLeon CM. Healing with Yagé: an interview with Taita Juan Bautista Agreda Chindoy. In: Therapeutic use of ayahuasca. Berlin: Springer; 2014. p. 197–215.
10. Coe, M. A Ethnomedical components of the ayahuasca complex: vegetalismo in the peruvian amazon region.B.S. Thesis. 2014, University of Hawaii at Mānoa.
11. Fotiou E. Working with "La Medicina": elements of healing in contemporary ayahuasca rituals. Anthropol Consciousness. 2012;23(1):6–27.
12. Riba J et al. Metabolism and disposition of N, N-dimethyltryptamine and harmala alkaloids after oral administration of ayahuasca. Drug TestingAnalysis. 2012;4(7–8):610–6.
13. Riba J et al. Human pharmacology of ayahuasca: subjective and cardiovascular effects, monoamine metabolite excretion, and pharmacokinetics. J PharmacolExp Ther. 2003;306(1): 73–83.
14. Riba J et al. Effects of the South American psychoactive beverage ayahuasca on regional brain electrical activity in humans: a functional neuroimaging study using low-resolution electromagnetic tomography. Neuropsychobiol. 2004;50(1):89–101.

15. McKenna DJ. The healing vine: ayahuasca as medicine in the 21st century. In: Winkelman MJ, Roberts TB, editors. Psychedelic medicine: New evidence for hallucinogenic substances as treatments. Westport: Praeger; 2007. p. 21–44.
16. Brierley D, Davidson C. Developments in harmine pharmacology: implications for ayahuasca use and drug-dependence treatment. Prog Neuropsychopharmacol Biol Psychiatry. 2012;39(2):263–72.
17. Luna LE. Vegetalismo: Shamanism among the Mestizo population of the Peruvian Amazon. Stockholm: Almqvist & Wiksell International; 1986.
18. Luna LE, Amaringo P. Ayahuasca visions: the religious iconography of a Peruvian shaman. Berkeley: North Atlantic Books; 1991.
19. Schultes RE, Hofmann A. Plants of the gods: their sacred, healing and hallucinogenic powers. Rochester: Healing Arts Press; 1992.
20. Luna LE. Ayahuasca shamanism shared across cultures. Cultural Survival Quarterly. 2003;27(2):20–3.
21. Tupper KW. Entheogenic healing: the spiritual effects and therapeutic potential of ceremonial ayahuasca use. In: Ellens JH, editor. The healing power of spirituality: how faith helps humans thrive. Westport: Praeger; 2009. p. 269–82.
22. Liester MB, Prickett J. Hypotheses regarding the mechanisms of ayahuasca in the treatment of addictions. J Psychoactive Drugs. 2012;44(3):200–8.
23. Luna LE. The concept of plants as teachers among four mestizo shamans of Iquitos, northeastern Peru. JEthnopharmacol. 1984;11(2):135–56.
24. Beyer SV. Special ayahuasca issue introduction: toward a multidisciplinary approach to ayahuasca studies. Anthropol Consciousness. 2012;23(1):1–5.
25. Winkleman MJ. Drug tourism or spiritual healing? Ayahuasca seekers in Amazonia. J Psychoactive Drugs. 2005;37(2):209–18.
26. Gerra G et al. Association between low-activity serotonin transporter genotype and heroin dependence: behavioral and personality correlates. Am J Med Genetics Part B Neuropsychiatric Genetics. 2004;126(1):37–42.
27. Hallikainen T et al. Association between low activity serotonin transporter promoter genotype and early onset alcoholism with habitual impulsive violent behavior. Molecular Psychiatry. 1999;4(4):385–8.
28. Mantere T et al. Serotonin transporter distribution and density in the cerebral cortex of alcoholic and nonalcoholic comparison subjects: a whole-hemisphere autoradiography study. Am J Psychiatry. 2014;159(4):599–606.
29. Callaway JC et al. Platelet serotonin uptake sites increased in drinkers of ayahuasca. Psychopharmacol. 1994;116(3):385–7.
30. Fernández X et al. Assessment of the psychotherapeutic effects of ritual ayahuasca use on drug dependence: a pilot study. In: The therapeutic use of ayahuasca. Berlin, Heidelberg: Springer; 2014. p. 183–96.
31. Osório FDL et al. Antidepressant effects of a single dose of ayahuasca in patients with recurrent depression: a preliminary report. Revista Brasileira de Psiquiatria. 2015;37(1):13–20.
32. de Lima Osório F et al. The therapeutic potential of harmine and ayahuasca in depression: evidence from exploratory animal and human studies. In: Santos RED, editor. The Ethnopharmacology of Ayahuasca. Trivandrum: Transworld Research Network; 2011.
33. Pacher P, Kecskemeti V. Trends in the development of new antidepressants. Is there a light at the end of the tunnel? Current Medicinal Chem. 2004;11(7):925.
34. Mabit J. Ayahuasca in the treatment of addictions. In: Winkelman MJ, Roberts TB, editors. Psychedelic medicine: new evidence for hallucinogenic substances as treatments. Westport: Praeger; 2007.
35. Winkleman MJ. Psychedelics as medicines for substance abuse rehabilitation: evaluating treatments with LSD, Peyote, Ibogaine and Ayahuasca. Current Drug Abuse Reviews. 2014;7(1):101–16.

36. Thomas G et al. Ayahuasca-assisted therapy for addictions: results from a preliminary observational study in Canada. Current Drug Abuse Reviews. 2013;6(1):30–42.
37. Labate BC et al. Effect of Santo Daime membership on substance dependence. In: The therapeutic use of ayahuasca. Berlin, Heidelberg: Springer; 2014. p. 153–9.
38. McKenna DJ. Ayahuasca: an ehtnopharmacologic history. In: Metzner R, editor. Ayahuasca: Hallucinogens, consciousness, and the spirit of nature. New York: Thunder's Mouth Press; 1999. p. 187–213.
39. Callaway JC. Ayahuasca preparations and serotonin reuptake inhibitors: a potential combination for severe adverse interactions. J Psychoactive Drugs. 1998;30(4):367–9.

Potential Herbal Anxiolytics

8

Erica McIntyre, David A. Camfield, and Jerome Sarris

8.1 Introduction

The herbal medicines described in this chapter are considered to be novel treatments for anxiety. While they have a long history of traditional use for a variety of medical conditions, they are not usually considered as treatments for anxiety, or are not commonly used outside of their native countries. These herbal treatments have been included, as they have been shown to possess some clinical evidence in human trials, and may be potential treatments for reducing symptoms of anxiety, although further research is required. The mechanisms of anxiolytic action for these herbs are yet to be firmly established, and it is recommended that future studies further investigate these substances in order to determine their efficacy in the treatment of anxiety. Table 8.1 provides a summary of these herbal medicines.

E. McIntyre (✉)
School of Psychology, Charles Sturt University, Bathurst, NSW, Australia

Faculty of Health, Australian Research Centre in Complementary and Integrative Medicine (ARCCIM), University of Technology, Ultimo, NSW, Australia
e-mail: emcintyre@csu.edu.au

D.A. Camfield
School of Psychology, University of Wollongong, Wollongong, NSW, Australia

Centre for Human Psychopharmacology, Swinburne University of Technology, Hawthorn, VIC, Australia

J. Sarris
University of Melbourne, Department of Psychiatry, The Melbourne Clinic, The Professorial Unit, ARCADIA Mental Health Research Group, 2 Salisbury St, Richmond, Melbourne, VIC 3121, Australia

Centre for Human Psychopharmacology, Swinburne University of Technology, Hawthorn, VIC, Australia

D. Camfield et al. (eds.), *Evidence-Based Herbal and Nutritional Treatments for Anxiety in Psychiatric Disorders*, DOI 10.1007/978-3-319-42307-4_8

Table 8.1 Summary of potential herbal anxiolytics

Herbal medicine	Dosage	Major/active constituents	Key evidence	Potential AEs	Potential clinical use	Clinical advice
Bitter orange (*Citrus aurantium*)	Acute dose: 1 ml/kg of distillate; standardized for linalool, total phenolic acids, and flavonoids. Administered 2 h prior to needing anxiolytic effect.	Limonene identified as having an anxiolytic effect in the serotonergic system via the $5HT_{1A}$ serotonin receptor.	One double-blind RCT demonstrating a reduction in postoperative anxiety.	Theoretical concerns about the pyrrolizidine alkaloid content in extract; however, studies to date have demonstrated no adverse effects.	For acute situational anxiety. Only has evidence for preoperative anxiety.	Distillate not recommended for long-term use. Not suitable for more chronic forms of anxiety. Anxiolytic effects of whole plant extracts are yet to be established. May have benefits for social anxiety, panic disorder, and anxiety related to specific phobias; however, research is needed to support this use.
Purple cone flower (*Echinacea angustifolia*)	Dried herb 3 g/day. Standardized for alkylamides.	Lipophilic alkylamides that bind to cannabinoid B1 receptors and regulate neurotransmitter function; are involved in GABA and glutamate modulation.	One RCT on healthy volunteers with elevated state and trait anxiety (treatment over 1 week). Demonstrated a reduction in both state and trait anxiety that was sustained over time (2 weeks post treatment).	Possible gastrointestinal side effects such as nausea, diarrhea, and stomach upset. Skin rash infrequently observed.	For generalized anxiety symptoms.	Promising initial evidence; however, more quality RCTs are needed. May have an adjunctive role in chronic forms of anxiety in which chronic stress-related immune responses occur.

Iranian borage (*Echium amoenum*)	Dried herb 1.1–1.6 g/day. No established standardization markers.	Yet to be established.	One clinical trial showing reduction in OCD and anxiety symptoms. One clinical trial showing an enhanced anxiolytic effect as adjunct with an SSRI. Traditional use in Iran.	No adverse reactions found in studies.	OCD and GAD. May be useful for generalized anxiety with mild to moderate depression.	May have an adjunctive role with SSRI treatment for GAD. Possible role to assist in withdrawal from SSRIs; however, more research is needed. May be difficult to source. Used traditionally as a tea. Standardization of low levels of pyrrolizidine alkaloids advised.
Milk thistle (*Silybum marianum*)	Dried seed 12–15 g/day in divided doses. Standardized to silymarin.	Yet to be established for anxiolytic and antiobsessive and anticompulsive effects. Possibly related to the flavonoid complex silymarin.	Minor research. Not supportive of anxiolytic effects. Weak evidence of efficacy for OCD symptoms. Some evidence of traditional use as an anxiolytic.	Generally considered safe. Mild digestive symptoms may be experienced, such as mild diarrhea.	Shows promise in the treatment of OCD and related disorders (i.e. trichotillomania). May be useful for generalized anxiety symptoms; however, more research is needed.	May have an adjunctive role in chronic forms of anxiety in which oxidative stress is involved.

8.2 Bitter Orange (*Citrus aurantium*)

8.2.1 Overview

Citrus aurantium is widely used throughout the world. Having originated in China, it has been used as a medicinal plant in traditional Chinese medicine for thousands of years [1]. Various plant parts (fruit, peel, leaves, bark, flowers) and preparations have been used for a wide range of conditions including: digestive complaints, respiratory infections, various psychological symptoms, and central nervous system disorders [1]. *Citrus aurantium* is reputed to have thermogenic, bronchospasmolytic, anticonvulsant, anxiolytic, and sedative actions [2]. The anxiolytic effects of *Citrus aurantium* have been demonstrated using the distilled essential oil from the peel as an aroma therapy treatment in clinical studies in a range of conditions [3–6]; however, clinical studies on the effects of whole plant extracts of *Citrus aurantium* have primarily focused on weight loss (as a herbal combination product), or assessing the safety of the herb—due to the presence of pyrrolizidine alkaloids [7]. Despite concerns about the pyrrolizidine alkaloid content in bitter orange extract, studies have demonstrated no adverse effects [7]; however, more research is needed.

8.2.2 Mechanisms of Action

The essential oil of *Citrus aurantium* has been shown to be responsible for anxiolytic effects, with the monoterpene limonene identified as the primary constituent responsible for this action [8]. The anxiolytic effect has been found to occur in the serotonergic system via the $5HT_{1A}$ serotonin receptor [8].

8.2.3 In Vivo Studies

Studies have demonstrated anxiolytic effects using the essential oil of *Citrus aurantium* in mice and rodents [9–11]; however, few studies have investigated these effects using whole plant extracts of bitter orange. One study on mice used the elevated plus maze (EPM) and the open-field test to investigate the anxiolytic effects of bitter orange in preparations of both the distilled essential oil from the peel and various hydroethanolic extracts of the leaves [2]. Mice were orally administered either essential oil (1 g/kg or 0.5 g/kg) or 1 g/kg of a hydroethanolic extract (crude extract, hexanic fraction, dichloromethanic fraction, aqueous fraction) or diazepam (1.2 mg/kg), or a control solution. Results revealed that only the essential oil and the diazepam groups significantly increased the number of entries into the open arms of the EPM compared to placebo, with the diazepam group demonstrating the greatest reduction in anxiety-like behaviors. No reduction in anxiety-like behaviors was observed for any treatment in the open-field test.

8.3 Evidence of Efficacy

8.3.1 Clinical Studies

The acute anxiolytic effects of bitter orange was assessed in a double-blind RCT [12]. Sixty preoperative patients ($n = 60$) with anxiety who were having a minor lower limb operation were randomized into two groups and orally administered either *Citrus aurantium* (blossom petals and stamens) distillate (1 ml/kg; standardized for linalool, total phenolic acids, and flavonoids); or placebo (saline solution 1 ml/kg). Treatments were administered 2 hours prior to the operation. Anxiety symptoms were measured using the State-Trait Anxiety Inventory (STAI)-state and the Amsterdam Preoperative Anxiety and Information Scale (APAIS), with physiological measures for heart rate and blood pressure at baseline (prior to treatments) and 2 hours later (directly before surgery). Patients in the bitter orange group demonstrated a significant reduction in anxiety scores on both the STAI-state and APAIS, while the placebo group did not show a significant reduction in anxiety. There were no significant differences in physiological measures for either group. However, the reporting of statistical results was problematic, with no group × time interaction stated. For this reason, it is difficult to establish whether reductions in anxiety observed in the bitter orange group were significantly greater than those observed in the placebo group.

8.4 Echinacea/Purple Cone Flower (*Echinacea* spp.)

8.4.1 Overview

Echinacea species are best known for their immunomodulatory and anti-inflammatory effects [13]. The flowers and roots of *Echinacea* spp. Have a long history of traditional use by indigenous North Americans who have used this medicine to treat a range of conditions including headaches, snake bite, toothache, and the common cold [14]. A variety of species have been used for their medicinal actions; however, *Echinacea purpurea, Echinacea angustifolia*, and *Echinacea pallida* species are most commonly used in modern herbal preparations [15]. The primary bioactive constituents in *Echinacea* spp. are alkylamides and polysaccharides, which are present at varying levels depending on the plant part used, with the roots having the greatest concentration of alkylamides [15].

8.4.2 Mechanisms of Action

The anxiolytic effect of *Echinacea* spp. may be due to a range of lipophilic alkylamide constituents that bind to cannabinoid B1 receptors predominantly located on neurons [13]. Cannabinoid B1 receptors regulate neurotransmitter function and are involved in GABA and glutamate modulation [16]. In addition, *E. angustifolia* extract has been demonstrated to reduce the release of glutamate and decrease synaptic excitation in the hippocampus; however, the specific constituents responsible for this action have not been identified [17].

8.4.3 In Vivo Studies

Two animal studies explored the anxiolytic activity of *Echinacea* spp. Anxiolytic-like effects were studied in rats using a variety of extraction types of either *E. purpurea* root, *E. purpurea* herb, or *E. angustifolia* root [18]. Various doses were tested depending on the extract used, and all doses were administered in a volume of 2 mL/kg. Three extracts decreased anxious behaviors to various degrees in the EPM, social interaction, and social avoidance tests. Significant anxiolytic effects were only observed at doses of 1.5 and 2 mg/kg for the *E. purpurea* root ethanol extract (4% echinacoside), 4 mg/kg for the *E. purpurea* root hydroalcohol extract (unstandardized), and 1 mg/kg for the *E. angustifolia* root ethanol extract (4 % echinacoside). Interestingly, the anxiolytic effects were not dose-dependently related to alkylamide content, although the three extracts demonstrating anxiolytic effects had considerably higher amounts of alkylamides compared to the ineffective extracts. Further investigation of the *E. angustifolia* extract found a dosage range of 3–6 mg/kg effective at 30 min following treatment, and 4–8 mg/kg at 1 hour after treatment. No locomotor-suppressant effects were seen for any extract at any dose.

A second study by the same group used the *E. angustifolia* extract from the previous study to investigate various behavioral effects including anxiolysis in rats [13]. They found a significant reduction in anxiety-like behaviors for the extract, with rats spending more time exploring open arms in the EPM, while displaying significantly reduced conditioned fear.

8.5 Evidence of Efficacy

8.5.1 Clinical Studies

The researchers from the above study conducted a RCT in 33 adults [13]. This clinical trial investigated the anxiolytic effects of *E. angustifolia* root (ethanol extract, 4 % echinacoside) in a healthy sample without a psychiatric diagnosis, but with high scores on the STAI (both state and trait). This was an open-label design with a 3-day observation phase, followed by a 1-week treatment phase and a 2-week washout period. Participants were randomly assigned to receive either one or two *E. angustifolia* tablets (20 mg extract) per day. Within 3 days, there was a significant decrease in both state and trait STAI scores for the higher dose of 40 mg per day that remained stable until day 7 (end of treatment) and for the 2-week follow-up observation period. No anxiolytic effect was found for the lower dose, and there were no serious adverse effects reported. Further research is needed using more robust methodology with a placebo comparison to support the use of *Echinacea* spp. in treating anxiety symptoms.

8.6 Iranian Borage (*Echium amoenum*)

8.6.1 Overview

Echium amoenum is an Iranian plant medicine with a long history of traditional use. The flowers and leaves have been used traditionally to treat heart disease, the common cold, and other pulmonary conditions [19]. The petals are used for their effects on the nervous system, as they have analgesic, anxiolytic, and sedative actions [19]. In traditional Iranian medicine, decoctions of the petals are consumed for the duration that the anxiety or stress symptoms are experienced [19], suggesting that this herbal medicine may be suitable for more chronic forms of anxiety. A range of constituents have been identified in the petals, which include saponins, flavonoids, unsaturated terpenoids, sterols [20], alkaloids (including pyrrolizidine alkaloids), and volatile oils [19, 21].

8.6.2 Mechanisms of Action

The mechanism of the anxiolytic action of *Echium amoenum* has yet to be firmly established. It is hypothesized that flavonoids may be responsible for the anxiolytic effect of *Echium amoenum* due to their ability to bind to benzodiazepine receptors [20].

8.6.3 In Vivo Studies

Five animal studies have investigated the anxiolytic effects of *Echium amoenum* flowers using either aqueous or hydroalcoholic extracts; with each type of extract demonstrating both acute and chronic anxiolytic-type effects [19–23]. For example, one study in mice explored both the acute and chronic anxiolytic effects of a hydroalcoholic extract of *Echium amoenum* flowers using the light/dark test [19]. Three doses (i.p.: 12.5, 25, and 50 mg/kg) were used and compared to diazepam and control treatments; each were administered as a single treatment for the acute test, and one dose per day for 1 week for the chronic test. Acute anxiolytic effects were found for 25 and 50 mg/kg *Echium amoenum* doses only, with mice spending significantly more time in the illuminated area. Chronic anxiolytic effects were found with 12.5, 25, and 50 mg/kg of the *Echium amoenum* extract per day over 1 week, with the greatest effect for the 50 mg dose. Anxiolytic effects were found for all active treatments with increased time spent in the illuminated zone, but not increased number of transitions.

8.7 Evidence of Efficacy

8.7.1 Clinical Studies

Two clinical trials to date have used an aqueous extract of *Echium amoenum* flowers to investigate the effects on chronic forms of anxiety. Forty-four patients with DSM-IV diagnosed OCD, and scores of 21 or over on the Yale-Brown Obsessive Compulsive Scale (Y-BOCS) were included in a 6-week, double-blind RCT investigating the efficacy and safety of Iranian borage [24]. Participants received either 500 mg/day of *Echium amoenum* (4 × 125 mg capsules) or placebo. Patients were assessed with the Y-BOCS and the Hamilton Anxiety Rating Scale (HAM-A) at baseline and weeks 1, 2, 4, and 6. A gradual reduction in OCD symptoms was observed for both groups, with a greater reduction in Y-BOCS for *Echium amoenum* compared to placebo at weeks 4 and 6 (6.27 point reduction in mean Y-BOCS scores at end point). A similar pattern was found for anxiety symptoms, with a significant reduction in HAM-A scores for *Echium amoenum* at weeks 4 and 6 (10.06 point reduction at end point), although this decrease was not significantly different than placebo. No significant difference in adverse effects was found between the two groups, although increased constipation was reported in the placebo group (talcum powder tablets).

Another RCT investigated the safety and efficacy of *Echium amoenum* flowers (aqueous extract) as a combined treatment with a selective-serotonin reuptake inhibitor (SSRI) for GAD [25]. Thirty-seven adults with DSM-IV-TR diagnosed GAD, and scores of 18 or more on the HAM-A were randomized into two groups receiving either *Echium amoenum* capsules (250 mg) three times daily plus fluoxetine (20 mg per day), or placebo capsules three times daily plus fluoxetine (20 mg per day). Adjunctive oxazepam (10 mg) was given in the case of insomnia. Participants were assessed using the HAM-A prior to treatment and at days 14, 28, 42, and 56 of treatment. *Echium amoenum* treatment was associated with greater reduction in HAMA-A scores compared to placebo, at both 14 and 56 days (study end point). No difference in the frequency of adverse events was found between groups, with headache being the most common side effect in the *Echium amoenum* group.

Sayyah and colleagues [26] also measured the anxiolytic effect of the same aqueous preparation of *Echium amoenum* in a double-blind RCT in adults ($n = 35$) with mild to moderate major depressive disorder (DSM-IV). Participants received either Iranian borage (1 × 125 mg capsule three times per day) or placebo capsules. Adjunctive oxazepam (5 mg) was given in the case of insomnia. Anxiety symptoms were measured with the HAM-A, and depression symptoms were measured with the Hamilton Rating Scale for Depression (HAM-D) at baseline and at 1, 2, 4, and 6 weeks of treatment. Changes in HAM-A scores across the 6 weeks were not significantly different between *Echium amoenum* and placebo; however, depressive symptoms gradually reduced over time and were significantly decreased at 4 weeks in comparison to placebo. The lower dose used in this study, together with a primarily depressed clinical group, may explain the nonsignificant result regarding anxiety.

8.7.2 Milk Thistle (*Silybum marianum*)

8.7.2.1 Overview

Silybum marianum has a long history of traditional use throughout Europe that dates back to biblical times [27]. Milk thistle also has a history of use in Chinese and Indian medicine, and is currently widely used throughout the world. It is best known for treating liver and gallbladder disorders; however, recent research has indicated its use as: an adjunctive treatment for certain cancers, diabetes and associated kidney disease, and neurodegenerative disorders [27, 28]. The American "eclectic" physicians Felter and Lloyd stated that milk thistle is specifically indicated for nervous irritability [29]. A recent ethnobotanical study in Iran found that the powdered seeds or stems of *Silybum marianum* is used by local traditional healers as a sedative [30].

The seed is the plant part most commonly used from *Silybum marianum,* containing flavonolignans (65–80 %), a flavonoid (taxifolin), fatty acids, and polyphenols. Extracts are usually standardized to silymarin (a complex including at least seven flavonolignans plus taxifolin) [31]. The predominant compound in silymarin is silibinin (containing silybin A and silybin B) [31]. Products used in clinical trials vary and may be *Silybum marianum* plant extracts, the silymarin complex, or silibinin. This is an important consideration when comparing the research and choosing the most appropriate herbal product. While milk thistle is not usually considered as a treatment for mental health conditions, its unique photochemistry suggests it may have beneficial effects on neurodegeneration and neurotransmitter function.

8.7.2.2 Mechanisms of Action

The mechanism of action for the reputed anti-OCD effects of *Silybum marianum* are unconfirmed; however, it may be attributed to the flavonoid complex silymarin, which in preclinical studies has been found to increase serotonin levels in the cortex [32], and prevent decreases in dopamine and serotonin in the prefrontal cortex and hippocampus related to methamphetamine use [33]. The increase in cortical serotonin levels and the resultant anti-obsessional effects may be attributable to silymarin inhibition of MAO activity as revealed by in vitro research [34]. Silymarin has also been found to interact with 5-HT_{1A} receptors in the serotonergic system [33, 35], as described in the following preclinical study.

8.8 Evidence of Efficacy

8.8.1 Preclinical

No preclinical studies presently exist, testing the whole plant extract of *Silybum marianum* to investigate anxiolytic effects; however, one study evaluated the anxiolytic effects of a silymarin complex using the EPM in rats [35]. This study also aimed to determine if silymarin interacted with 5-HT_{1A} receptors. A series of animal model experiments were conducted that compared various doses of silymarin (p.o.), with a 5-HT receptor agonist (i.c.v.), a 5-HT receptor antagonist (i.c.v.), and placebo (p.o.ori.c.v.) over 2 weeks. Results showed that oral doses of 35, 70, and 140 mg per rat (180–230 g) over 2 weeks significantly reduced anxiety behaviors, with an increase in time spent in the open arms and in the number of entries in open arms of the EPM, with similar effects found for the 5-HT_{1A} receptor agonist. The 5-HT_{1A} receptor antagonist significantly decreased both entries into and time spent in the open arms. Significantly increased anxiolytic effects were observed when silymarin was administered prior to the 5-HT_{1A} agonist, which contrasted with reduced anxiolytic effects for silymarin when the 5-HT_{1A} antagonist was administered. The authors concluded that 5-HT_{1A} receptors are involved in the anxiolytic effects of silymarin.

8.9 Evidence of Efficacy

8.9.1 Clinical Studies

A double-blind, RCT compared the effects of fluoxetine to *Silybum marianum* leaf extract (methanol) in 35 adults with a DSM-IV diagnosis of OCD and a score of 21 or greater on the Y-BOCS, which indicates moderate–severe OCD [36]. Participants received capsules of either 200 mg of *Silybum marianum* extract (standardization and chemical profile not disclosed) or 10 mg of fluoxetine, three times daily for 8 weeks. Adjunctive oxazepam (10 mg) was given in the case of insomnia. Significant reductions in Y-BOCS scores were found for both fluoxetine and *Silybum marianum* over the 8-week period. However, the Y-BOCS reduction observed for *Silybum marianum* at study end point was not significantly different than that observed for fluoxetine. These results suggest that *Silybum marianum* may be equally as effective as fluoxetine in reducing obsessive compulsive symptoms; however, a slightly delayed effect was observed for *Silybum marianum* (with reductions not observed until week 1). It is also noteworthy that in this study, baseline Y-BOCS scores were particularly high, and without a placebo group it is difficult to determine to what extent the decreases were due to the active substances administered.

A double-blind, placebo-controlled, crossover study in patients with hepatitis C virus (HCV; $n = 24$) measured the effects of *Silybum marianum* seed extract (standardized to 80 % silymarin) on anxiety symptoms and general mental health, in addition to physiological indicators of HCV [37]. Over a 12-week period, patients received a single daily dose of either 600 or 1200 mg tablets or placebo, with a washout period of 4 weeks between treatments. State anxiety and general mental health were assessed using the STAI-S and Short Form-36 Health Survey (SF-36), respectively, at baseline, end of treatment, and 12 weeks following treatment. *Silybum marianum* treatments were not found to significantly reduce SF-36 or STAI-S scores at end point; however, there was a significantly greater decrease in anxiety for placebo. The reason for the reduction due to placebo (and not milk thistle) in this study is unclear; it is possible that milk thistle is better suited to specific types of anxiety-related disorders such as OCD.

Of interest, three brief case studies were published that described the effectiveness of silymarin in reducing obsessive and compulsive symptoms [38]. In one female patient with trichotillomania of moderate severity (National Institute of Mental Health Trichotillomania Symptom Severity scale), a reduction in symptoms was observed after 6 weeks of treatment (150 mg twice daily), with near cessation of symptoms reported after 4 months. In the second case, a woman with OCD of moderate severity demonstrated a 10-point reduction in Y-BOCS scores after 8 weeks of treatment with 300 mg silymarin twice daily. For the third case, a male patient showed a reduction in nail-biting symptoms (clinical observation) following 4 weeks of treatment (150 mg per day). The patient stopped treatment soon after this; however, 2 weeks later, the nail-biting symptoms returned to pretreatment severity. Symptoms resolved again following an additional 4 weeks of treatment. No side effects were reported by these patients.

Given the findings reported, more research is needed to confirm the efficacy of *Silybum marianum* in treating anxiety symptoms and obsessive–compulsive symptoms. Case study observations suggest that future research could focus on obsessive–compulsive symptoms.

8.10 Clinical Considerations

The four herbs covered in this chapter have shown preliminary evidence for treating anxiety or obsessive–compulsive symptoms, despite not usually being considered for this indication. Specifically, *Echium amoenum* was effective in reducing anxiety and obsessive–compulsive symptoms in OCD, while *Silybum marianum* demonstrated a significant improvement in OCD symptoms, but not anxiety symptoms. *Citrus aurantium* demonstrated acute anxiolytic effects in preoperative anxiety, and *Echinacea angustifolia* was found to reduce both state and trait anxiety in healthy adults.

Given that *Echinacea angustifolia* has a good safety profile [39], and its anxiolytic effects were sustained over a period of time, it is worthy of consideration in more chronic forms of anxiety. In addition, a relatively rapid reduction in anxiety (significant at day 3 of treatment) was found for *Echinacea* that was comparable to diazepam; however, this effect needs to be evaluated in more severe anxiety disorders [13]. As *Echium amoenum* has been demonstrated to reduce anxiety symptoms gradually over time, this herb would be most suitable for use in more chronic cases of clinically significant anxiety, such as OCD and GAD, which aligns with its traditional use in Iranian herbal medicine. Iranian borage may also be considered when there is comorbid depression. Correct dosage needs to be considered, as significant anxiolytic effects were not found at lower doses, and higher doses may have an unwanted sedative effect. Further, as this plant contains hepatotoxic pyrrolizidine alkaloids, preparations must standardize for low levels of this compound. *Citrus aurantium* may be suitable for use in preventing acute anxiety related to social anxiety and other types of situational anxiety.

All herbs discussed in this section have a relatively good safety profile; however, more research is needed to establish safety in longer term use and to determine potential herb–drug interactions. *Echium amoenum* was found to be a safe adjunctive treatment with an SSRI. Theoretically, this herb could be considered to either enhance the effects of SSRIs or assist in SSRI withdrawal. In addition, these herbs may be useful when combined with other herbal anxiolytics with more established efficacy such as *Piper methysticum* and *Passiflora incarnata*. When selecting the most suitable herbal medicine, individual patient characteristics need to be considered. For example, due to its antioxidant properties, *Silybum marianum* may be indicated when there is oxidative stress associated with more chronic disorders such as OCD; and *Echinacea* may be suitable when there is chronic stress-related immune responses occurring [39].

Some of the studies discussed do not use clearly established standardized, chemically defined extracts (e.g. Iranian borage, milk thistle). The lack of phytoequivalence between extracts prevents the advancement of knowledge regarding the anxiolytic properties of botanicals as viable alternatives to pharmaceuticals. This problem could be resolved if appropriate information regarding the exact quantities of active constituents was provided in future articles reporting clinical studies. In addition, chemical composition of herbal preparation depends on many factors, such as genetic and environmental differences, exposure to airborne vectors, differences in plant parts used, harvest time, and preparation methods. The application of analytic and "omic" (e.g. genomic, proteomic, metabolomic) technology would greatly assist in providing assurance of bioequivalence [40, 41].

While the herbs discussed in this chapter have demonstrated some evidence of anxiolytic effects, more research is needed to clearly establish their safety and efficacy in chronic and acute anxiety, for obsessive and compulsive symptoms, and as adjuncts to psychological and pharmaceutical treatments. Theoretically, these herbs may be useful when combined with other herbal anxiolytics when their established primary therapeutic actions are indicated.

References

1. Paul A, Cox PA. An ethnobotanical survey of the uses for Citrus aurantium (Rutaceae) in Haiti. Econ Bot. 1995;49(3):249–56.
2. Carvalho-Freitas MIR, Costa M. Anxiolytic and sedative effects of extracts and essential oil from *Citrus Aurantium* L. Biol Pharm Bull. 2002;25(12):1629–33.
3. Goes TC, Antunes FD, Alves PB, Teixeira-Silva F. Effect of sweet orange aroma on experimental anxiety in humans. J Altern Complement Med. 2012;18(8):798–804.
4. Namazi M, Akbari SAA, Mojab F, Talebi A, Majd HA, Jannesaria S. Effects of *Citrus Aurantium* (Bitter Orange) on the severity of first-stage labor pain. Iran J Pharm Res. 2014;13(3):1011–8.
5. Namazi M, Amir Ali Akbari S, Mojab F, Talebi A, Alavi Majd H, Jannesari S. Aromatherapy with Citrus aurantium oil and anxiety during the first stage of labor. Iran Red Crescent Med J. 2014;16(6):e18371.
6. Cho MY, Min ES, Hur MH, Lee MS. Effects of aromatherapy on the anxiety, vital signs, and sleep quality of percutaneous coronary intervention patients in intensive care units. Evid Based Complement Alternat Med eCAM. 2013;2013:381381.

7. Stohs SJ, Preuss HG, Shara M. A review of the human clinical studies involving Citrus aurantium (bitter orange) extract and its primary protoalkaloid p-synephrine. Int J Med Sci. 2012;9(7):527–38.
8. Costa CA, Cury TC, Cassettari BO, Takahira RK, Flório JC, Costa M. Citrus aurantium L. essential oil exhibits anxiolytic- like activity mediated by 5-HT1A-receptors andreduces cholesterol after repeated oral treatment. BMC Complementary Altern Med. 2013;13(42):1–10.
9. Pultrini Ade M, Galindo LA, Costa M. Effects of the essential oil from Citrus aurantium L. in experimental anxiety models in mice. Life Sci. 2006;78(15):1720–5.
10. Leite MP, Fassin Jr J, Baziloni F, Almeida RN, Mattei R, Leite JR. Behavioral effects of essential oil of *Citrus aurantium* L. inhalation in rats. Braz J Pharmacognosy. 2008;18(Supp): 661–6.
11. Khosravi M, Khakpour S, Adibi L, Jahromy MH. A study of the effect of *Citrus aurantium* L. essential oil on anxiety and its interaction with GABAergic pathways in male mice. J Behav Brain Sci. 2014;04(10):470–6.
12. Akhlaghi M, Shabanian G, Rafieian-Kopaei M, Parvin N, Saadat M. Citrus aurantium blossom and preoperative anxiety. RevBrasAnestesiol. 2011;61(6):702–12.
13. Haller J, Freund TF, Pelczer KG, Furedi J, Krecsak L, Zambori J. The anxiolytic potential and psychotropic side effects of an echinacea preparation in laboratory animals and healthy volunteers. Phytother Res. 2013;27(1):54–61.
14. Kindscher K. Ethnobotany of purple coneflower (Echinacea angustifolia, Astraceae) and other echinacea species. Econ Bot. 1989;43(4):498–507.
15. Woelkart K, Baur R. The role of alkamides as an active principle of echinacea. Planta Med. 2007;73:615–23.
16. Tambaro S, Bortolato M. Cannabinoid-related agents in the treatment of anxiety disorders: current knowledge and future perspectives. CNS Drugs Discov. 2012;7(1):25–40.
17. Hájos N, Holderith N, Németh B, Papp OI, Szabó GG, Zemankovics R, et al. The effects of an echinacea preparation on synaptic transmission and the firing properties of CA1 pyramidal cells in the hippocampus. Phytother Res. 2012;26(3):354–62.
18. Haller J, Hohmann J, Freund TF. The effect of Echinacea preparations in three laboratory tests of anxiety: comparison with chlordiazepoxide. Phytother Res. 2010;24(11):1605–13.
19. Rabbani M, Sajjadi SE, Khalili S. A lack of tolerance to the anxiolytic action of Echium amoenum. Res Pharm Sci. 2011;6(2):101–6.
20. Gholamzadeh S, Zare S, Ikhanipoor M. Anxiolytic effect of Echium amoenum during different treatment courses. Res Biol Sci. 2008;3(2):176–8.
21. Gholamzadeh S, Zare S, Ilkhanipoor M. Evaluation of the anxiolytic effect of Echium amoenum petalsextract, during chronic treatment in rat. Res Pharm Sci. 2007;2(2):91–5.
22. Rabbani M, Sajjadi SE, Vaseghi G, Jafarian A. Anxiolytic effects of Echium amoenum on the elevated plus-maze model of anxiety in mice. Fitoterapia. 2004;75(5):457–64.
23. Shafaghi B, Naderi N, Tahmasb L, Kamalinejad M. Anxiolytic effect of Echium amoenum L. in Mice. Iran J Pharm Res. 2002;1:37–41.
24. Sayyah M, Boostani H, Pakseresht S, Malaieri A. Efficacy of aqueous extract of Echium amoenum in treatment of obsessive-compulsive disorder. Prog Neuropsychopharmacol Biol Psychiatry. 2009;33(8):1513–6.
25. Sayyah M, Siahpoosh A, Khalili H, Malaieri A, Samaee H. A double-blind, placebo-controlled study of the aqueous extract ofEchium amoenum for patients with general anxiety disorder. Iran J Pharm Res. 2012;11(2):697–701.
26. Sayyah M, Sayyah M, Kamalinejad M. A preliminary randomized double blind clinical trial on the efficacy ofaqueous extract of Echium amoenum in the treatment of mild to moderatemajor depression. Prog Neuro-Psychopharmacol Biol Psychiatry. 2006;30:166–9.
27. Abenavoli L, Capasso R, Milic N, Capasso F. Milk thistle in liver diseases: past, present, future. Phytother Res. 2010;24(10):1423–32.
28. Bahmani M, Shirzad H, Rafieian S, Rafieian-Kopaei M. Silybum marianum: beyond Hepatoprotection. J Evid Based Complementary Altern Med. 2015;20(4):292–301.

29. Felter HW, Lloyd JU. King's American dispensatory. 1898.
30. Mosaddegh M, Naghibi F, Moazzeni H, Pirani A, Esmaeili S. Ethnobotanical survey of herbal remedies traditionally used in Kohghiluyeh va Boyer Ahmad province of Iran. J Ethnopharmacol. 2012;141(1):80–95.
31. Kroll DJ, Shaw HS, Oberlies NH. Milk thistle nomenclature: why it matters in cancer research and pharmacokinetic studies. Integr Cancer Ther. 2007;6(2):110–9.
32. Osuchowski MF, Johnson VJ, He Q, Sharma RP. Alterations in regional brain neurotransmitters by silymarin, a natural antioxidant flavonoid mixture, in BALB/c mice. Pharmaceutical Biol. 2004;42(4–5):384–9.
33. Lu P, Mamiya T, Lu L, Mouri A, Niwa M, Kim HC, et al. Silibinin attenuates cognitive deficits and decreases of dopamine and serotonin induced by repeated methamphetamine treatment. Behav Brain Res. 2010;207(2):387–93.
34. Mazzio EA, Harris N, Soliman KFA. Food constituents attenuate monoamine oxidase activity and peroxide levels in C6 astrocyte cells. Planta Medica. 1998;64(7):603–6.
35. Solati J, Yaghmaei P, Mohammdadi K. Role of the 5-HT1A serotonergic system in anxiolytic-like effects of Silymarin. Neurophysiol. 2012;44(1):49–55.
36. Sayyah M, Boostani H, Pakseresht S, Malayeri A. Comparison of Silybum marianum (L.) Gaertn. with fluoxetine in the treatment of obsessive–compulsive disorder. Prog Neuro-Psychopharmacol Biol Psychiatry. 2010;34(2):362–5.
37. Gordon A, Hobbs DA, Bowden DS, Bailey MJ, Mitchell J, Francis AJP, et al. Effects of Silybum marianum on serum hepatitis C virus RNA, alanine aminotransferase levels and well-being in patients with chronic hepatitis C. J Gastroenterol Hepatol. 2006;21(1):275–80.
38. Grant JE, Odlaug BL. Silymarin treatment of obsessive-compulsive spectrum disorders. J Clin Psychopharmacol. 2015;35(3):340–2.
39. Ardjomand-Woelkart K, Bauer R. Review and assessment of medicinal safety data of orally used *Echinacea* preparations. Planta Medica. 2016;82(01/02):17–31.
40. Sarris J, Ng C, Schweitzer I. "Omic" genetic technologies for herbal medicines in psychiatry. Phytother Res. 2011;26:522–7.
41. Ulrich-Merzenich G, Zeitler H, Jobst D, Panek D, Vetter H, Wagner H. Application of the "-Omic-" technologies in phytomedicine. Phytomedicine. 2007;14(1):70–82.

Part III

Clinical Perspectives and Case Studies

9 Integrative Treatments for Masked Anxiety and PTSD in Highly Sensitive Patients

Patricia L. Gerbarg and Richard P. Brown

9.1 Introduction

Although anxiety is not always the most obvious symptom in complex cases, it must be recognized and addressed. The following four cases represent unrecognized atypical presentations of anxiety disorders and posttraumatic stress disorder (PTSD) in patients who did not respond well to conventional psychotropic medications. In these cases, affective, cognitive, and behavioral symptoms significantly improved with integrative treatments combining medicinal herbs, nootropics, other complementary approaches, and in some cases prescription psychotropic medications. When stress-related physical symptoms, such as dystonias, become the focus of treatment, the anxiety underlying the physical condition may escape notice. Patients who do not respond well to conventional medications or who have drug sensitivities are often mislabeled as "treatment-resistant." The urgent need for behavioral control of patients with developmental disorders, learning disabilities, and communication impairments often leads to the overuse of sedating major tranquilizers that miss the real target symptoms and exacerbate underlying cognitive and coordination dysfunctions. The treatment of anxiety, depression, and mild cognitive impairment in elderly patients with mild herbal formulas can significantly improve quality of life. Patients who do not respond adequately to prescription psychotropics and those who are sensitive to medication side effects are a large subgroup of people who benefit most from integrative and complementary approaches.

P.L. Gerbarg, MD (✉)
New York Medical College, Valhalla, NY, USA
e-mail: PGerbarg@aol.com; http://www.Breath-Body-Mind.com

R.P. Brown, MD
Columbia University College of Medicine, New York, NY, USA

D. Camfield et al. (eds.), *Evidence-Based Herbal and Nutritional Treatments for Anxiety in Psychiatric Disorders*, DOI 10.1007/978-3-319-42307-4_9

9.2 Clinical Cases

9.2.1 Case #1 Stress and Cervical Dystonia

9.2.1.1 Presenting Complaint

Eleanor, a 42-year-old dental assistant had suffered from cervical dystonia, a neurological condition characterized by painful involuntary chronic contractions or spasm of the neck muscles. Hers was mainly on the right side causing difficulty turning her head to the left. When Eleanor told her doctor that the dystonia was exacerbated by stress, she was treated with benzodiazepines, including clonazepam (Klonopin), alprazolam (Xanax), and lorazepam (Ativan). They all made her groggy and cognitively impaired. Trials of antidepressants, including fluoxetine (Prozac), sertraline (Zoloft), paroxetine (Paxil), and desipramine (Norpramine) failed to provide relief and made her jittery.

During the previous 18 months, Eleanor's symptoms became increasingly severe. She consulted a neurologist who administered Botulinum toxin B (botox) injections into the neck muscles without any effect. Botox injections are used in the treatment of dystonias, including cervical dystonia. The toxins inhibit acetylcholine release from neuromuscular junctions, producing muscle weakness and relaxation when injected into dystonic muscles. Next, the neurologist thought that she had an unusual variant of Parkinson's disease and treated her with trihexyphenidyl (Artane).This gave no benefit, but caused anticholinergic side effects of memory impairment, dry mouth, blurred vision, and constipation.

9.2.1.2 Diagnosis and Treatment Plan

Eleanor pursued a course in yoga breathing, which she found somewhat relaxing. Through this program, she heard about an integrative psychiatrist and contacted him for an evaluation. Looking beyond the physical manifestation of the cervical dystonia, the psychiatrist elicited a history of constant worrying, difficulty sleeping, recurrent worries while dreaming, difficulty making decisions, and other indicators of autonomic dysfunction, such as feeling too hot or too cold. He concluded that her underlying diagnosis was generalized anxiety disorder (GAD). Knowing from the patient's history that she was highly sensitive to medication side effects, a combination of *Melissa officinalis* (lemon balm) and L-theanine was prescribed. Lemon balm has been shown to relieve mild anxiety, provide mild sedation, and lessen drug withdrawal syndromes [1]. L-theanine is an amino acid (L-γ-glutamylethylamide or n-ethylglutamic acid) found in green and black teas made from *Camellia sinensis*. Studies demonstrate that L-theanine is mildly calming and is associated with a cortical alpha-pattern, indicative of a state of relaxed alertness [2]. Mechanisms of action include upregulation of inhibitory neurotransmitters, possible modulation of serotonin and dopamine in selected areas, increased levels of brain-derived neurotrophic factor, and neuroprotective effects [3]. Lemon balm 500 mg (Full Spectrum Lemon Balm, Swanson's) plus L-theanine (SunTheanine) 200 mg (Theanine 200, Jarrow) were prescribed three times a day. These caused no side effects.

9.2.1.3 Treatment Outcome

After 1 month of this treatment, Eleanor reported a marked improvement in her dystonia. In order to further empower the patient's own abilities to prevent stress from increasing muscle tension in her body, she was referred for a course of guided imagery and energy work. Through this approach and ongoing use of lemon balm and L-theanine, she stabilized, and the dystonia resolved. During the past 7 years, she has improved such that she only uses the lemon balm and L-theanine intermittently when under stress.

9.2.1.4 Discussion

The key to this case was recognizing the connection between muscle tension/spasm and chronic anxiety. That the patient herself sensed this and that she found a physician who listened to her self-observations made all the difference. The second key was acknowledging her sensitivity to side effects and combining two mildly calming herbal treatments with low side-effect profiles. When using phytomedicines with gentle effects for patients who have severe anxiety-related symptoms, it is often necessary to combine two or more herbal treatments in order to obtain a clinically meaningful response.

9.2.2 Case #2 Posttraumatic Stress Disorder Hidden by a Cosmetic Life

9.2.2.1 Presenting Complaint

Samantha, a 29-year-old socialite, had exquisite taste in clothes, accessories, and jewelry. Always an excellent athlete, she glided into the office on her 5-inch heels, extended her hand in greeting, and announced, "On paper I have a great life." She seemed animated and vivacious, but insisted that she was depressed. She was able to occupy one of the chairs for about a minute before she began pacing incessantly while wringing her hands and nervously smoothing her skirt. Her face remained apprehensive as she recounted the list of anxiolytics and antidepressants that had failed to bring her any relief: alprazolam (Xanax), clonazepam (Klonopin), buspirone (Buspar), zolpidem (Ambien), sertraline (Zoloft), escitalopram (Lexapro), venlafaxine (Effexor), aripiprazole (Abilify), lamotrigine (Lamictal), and gabapentin (Neurontin). Mirtazapine (Remeron) had helped a little, but she discontinued it after gaining 20 pounds in 1 month. She had tolerated a subtherapeutic dose of S-adenosylmethionine (SAMe) 600 mg/day.

Samantha's mother developed ovarian cancer when she was 2 years old and died when she was 12. When she was 5, her parents divorced. Samantha saw her father intermittently until after her mother's death. She was diagnosed as having irritable bowel syndrome at age 12 when she began to live with him. He was an angry, irritable man, an alcoholic, who could be frightening, but was not physically abusive. Following the World Trade Center attacks on September 11, 2001, Samantha developed a morbid fear of terrorists. She saw numerous doctors, who prescribed the medications listed above. Previous therapists who had treated her for anxiety and depression commented in their referral notes, "This is the most anxious patient I have ever seen." Hoping to have children, Samantha married a man who was 15 years older than she was. Shortly after the marriage, she developed morbid fears of nausea and vomiting during pregnancy, of having children, and of dying from uterine cancer like her mother. Her husband proved to be emotionally abusive and intolerant of her anxiety. After 4 months, they divorced.

9.2.2.2 Diagnosis and Treatment Plan

The integrative psychiatrist considered her primary diagnosis to be PTSD stemming from the trauma of having a mother dying of cancer at home during most of her childhood, losing her mother at age 12, and living with a difficult father. In addition, she met criteria for GAD, panic disorder, and dysthymic disorder. By history, she was highly sensitive to psychotropic side effects and treatment-resistant to synthetic anxiolytics and antidepressants.

Samantha entered treatment on stable doses of clonazepam 1.0 mg daily and SAMe 600 mg in the morning. In order to reduce anxiety and insomnia, she was treated for 20 min twice a day with cranial electrotherapy stimulation (CES) using a small home unit (level-2, Fischer Wallace-100). Cranial electrotherapy stimulation is a noninvasive electromedical treatment approved by the US Food and Drug Administration that emits a weak pulsed current (<4 milliamps) via electrodes placed on the temples or ear lobes. Numerous studies have shown benefits for anxiety, insomnia, and depression [4]. Samantha responded to CES with modest improvements in both anxiety and sleep.

Samantha was then given a trial of 25 mg/day of 7-keto DHEA (dehydroepiandrosterone), which has been reported to ameliorate symptoms of PTSD in case studies [5]. 7-keto DHEA is a neurohormone related to DHEA. Low levels of DHEA have been associated with vulnerability to PTSD [6]. Unfortunately, she reacted with increased anxiety, shakiness, and tearfulness. Such reactions are more common in patients with bipolar conditions, but neither she nor her family had a history of bipolar disorder.

The patient wanted to discontinue all prescription medications and tried to withdraw herself from clonazepam. Subsequently, she complained of feeling unwell, weak, and shaky—symptoms of benzodiazepine withdrawal. A course of 10–20 mg/day baclofen (Lioresal) alleviated the withdrawal symptoms. Attempting to treat the depression, she was prescribed *Crocus sativus L.* (saffron), which is a herb known to be low in side effects [7, 8] (optimized saffron with Satiereal, Life Extension Foundation), starting with a 88.25 mg capsule (standardized to 0.3 % safranal, 0.265 mg) twice a day and increasing to two capsules twice a day. Samantha tolerated saffron and found it to be mildly helpful for depression. Antidepressant effects of saffron have been demonstrated in clinical trials [9].

The PTSD was treated with *Withania somnifera* (Ashwaganda), an adaptogenic herb, in order to reduce anxiety and improve stress resilience [10]. Ashwaganda (Tranquility Kare, Kare-N-Herbs) was chosen because, among the adaptogenic herbs, it is particularly calming and is least likely to cause stimulation, agitation, or anxiety. The initial dose, 200 mg/day, was increased over 2 weeks to 400 mg three times a day. For the first time, Samantha reported significant relief of anxiety, subjectively about 50 % improvement.

Subsequently, increasing the morning dose of SAMe to 800 mg further relieved the depression. Over the next 6 weeks, SAMe was gradually increased to 1200 mg/day with additional improvement in depression symptoms. Treatment trials continued in an attempt to augment the anxiolytic and antidepressant effects that had occurred. Tianeptine (Stablon), an antidepressant with relatively few side effects [11], is a serotonin uptake accelerator (opposite action to serotonin reuptake inhibitors, SSRIs), and it does not cause sexual dysfunction or weight gain [12, 13]. In animal models, it reduces symptoms related to PTSD, an effect not seen with fluoxetine [14]. Nevertheless, when a starting dose of 100 mg Stablon exacerbated Samantha's anxiety and obsessive thoughts about aging and dying, it was discontinued.

Gamma-aminobutyric acid (GABA) is the primary inhibitory neurotransmitter in the brain. Normal levels of GABA-ergic activity are necessary to inhibit over-reactivity in the amygdala within the limbic system, where emotions, including fear and anger, are processed [15]. In PTSD, underactivation of GABA-ergic pathways can lead to failure to inhibit intense, trauma-related reactions, allowing more symptoms to occur [15]. Considering PTSD to be the underlying cause of Samantha's insomnia and anxiety, she was given a trial of 500 mg of GABA (GABA, Swanson) at bedtime. The GABA enabled her to reduce nighttime worry, fall asleep more quickly, sleep more hours, experience fewer anxiety dreams, obtain restorative sleep, and feel better the next day [16].

9.2.2.3 Treatment Outcome

Samantha feels better than she had in years on the combination of SAMe 1600 mg a day, ashwaganda 400 mg three times a day, saffron 176.5 mg a day, and GABA 500 mg at night. She had been referred previously for eye movement desensitization and reprocessing (EMDR) to help resolve more of the trauma-related problems. At that time, she and the therapist felt she could not tolerate the anxiety that could be provoked during EMDR. However, now that she feels better, she is restarting and tolerating EMDR.

9.2.2.4 Discussion

As in the previous case, it was of critical importance to find treatments that this sensitive patient could tolerate and then layer one upon another to augment the modest benefits of each treatment. The trial of ashwaganda, which is generally well tolerated, was pivotal in shifting the patient's nervous system to a place of significantly reduced over-reactivity, which ameliorated both her anxiety and insomnia. Adaptogens increase stress resilience and improve autonomic nervous system balance, thereby reducing anxiety, agitation, and over-reactivity.

9.2.3 Case #3 Anxiety Masked by Developmental Disorders

9.2.3.1 Presenting Complaint

After a 9-month inpatient hospitalization for severe violent attacks on her family and caregivers, Myra's family brought her for consultation, because they were worried about managing their 10-year-old at home. She had been in and out of hospitals since the age of 7, and had been hospitalized and evaluated at several leading academic centers. Myra had multiple nonverbal learning disabilities and had been given numerous developmental disorder diagnoses, including autism spectrum disorder and Asperger's. Furthermore, due to an articulation disorder, her speech was almost incomprehensible.

During her many hospitalizations, she had been given trials of antipsychotics, sedative hypnotics, mood stabilizers, and antidepressants alone and in combinations, including clonazepam (Klonopin), risperdone (Rispidal), olanzapine (Zyprexa), quetiapine (Seroquel), aripiprazole (Abilify), valproate (Depakote), carbamazepine (Tegratol), lithium carbonate (LithoBid), lamotrigine (Lamictal), fluoxetine (Prozac), sertraline (Zoloft), paroxetine (Paxil), and venlafaxine (Effexor). Some of the medications made her sedated or groggy, but none were effective in controlling her violent outbursts. She had gained 80 pounds on psychotropic medications. Since entering puberty, the violence escalated during the week prior to menses.

9.2.3.2 Diagnosis and Treatment Plan

The patient's diagnoses included autism spectrum disorder (ASD) (previously pervasive developmental disorder), bipolar disorder (which occurs at a high rate in ASD), speech sound disorder (phonological disorder), and intermittent explosive disorder.

In order to improve mood and reduce rage and aggression, Myra was started on ziprasidone (Geodon) 20 mg/day, and over a period of 2 months, increased to 80 mg twice a day. Ziprasidone was chosen because it is less sedating and less likely to cause weight gain. She tolerated ziprasidone and showed modest improvement in her mood and rage; however, the violent outbursts continued.

After 3 months, the patient was given a trial of piracetam, one of the pyrrolidone nootropics that have been shown to improve speech in patients with poststroke aphasia and in children with dyslexia [17, 18]. Piracetam, a derivative of the neurotransmitter GABA, restores cell membrane fluidity, modulates neurotransmission, has neuroprotective and anticonvulsant effects, and enhances neuroplasticity [19]. She began to improve by 4 weeks in response to piracetam, with a marked improvement in articulation over a 3-month period. Once her speech became more intelligible, her ability to communicate with her family and caregivers improved. She was better able to communicate her needs without becoming frustrated. Her caregivers were able to respond more effectively once they could understand what she was saying. She was able to benefit more from home schooling.

It became clearer that anxiety was driving Myra's mental and physical agitation. Lemon balm (*Melissa officinalis*), used on an as-needed (prn) basis, significantly relieved her anxiety and agitation within 1 week based on clinical global improvement and her mother's report. She learned how to request it when she noticed herself becoming upset or agitated. This enabled her, for the first time in her life, to regulate her own emotions. For the first time, she was able to live at home during the summer instead of being hospitalized. She continued to experience premenstrual exacerbations. These decreased when she was treated with Femaprin Vitex Extract,

(Nature's Way) two capsules per day, each capsule containing 225 mg *Vitex agnus-castus* (chaste tree) fruit extract standardized to 0.6 % agnusides, 100 mg *Vitex agnus-castus* fruit, and 100 mg vitamin B6 pyridoxine.

After being on ziprasidone for 4 years, Myra developed a massive neck dystonia, severe muscle spasm, and oral dyskinesias (abnormal repetitive movements of the mouth). The ziprasidone was discontinued and replaced with 3.75 mg/day of olanzapine (Zyprexa). Three months later, she was put on 100 mg twice a day of amantadine (Symmetrel) to prevent weight gain from the olanzapine [20].

9.2.3.3 Discussion

The challenges in this case were to clarify the diagnosis, to identify the treatable symptoms, and to find effective treatments that would not cause intolerable side effects. The treatment steps were as follows:

1. Find a tolerable medication with antipsychotic and anxiolytic effects that would not cause sedation, grogginess, or weight gain.
2. Address the speech disorder, so that the patient would be able to communicate.
3. Alleviate the underlying anxiety and agitation. Give the patient a means to regulate her emotions.
4. Relieve the premenstrual syndrome exacerbations.

The prescribed combination treatment of an antipsychotic (ziprasidone), a nootropic (piracetam), a calming herb (lemon balm), and a mild phytoestrogen (chaste tree) enabled Myra to live at home, avoid rehospitalization, receive home schooling, communicate with her family and caregivers, and gain confidence in her ability to control her own emotional reactions.

9.2.4 Case #4 Anxiety in the Guise of a Dementia

9.2.4.1 Presenting Complaint

Marvin, a 91-year-old Holocaust survivor, had been living in South America until his wife died 10 years ago, at which time he had moved to Philadelphia to be near his family. Marvin had remained active, taking long walks every day and practicing Tai Chi. Nevertheless, as he got older and began having more physical problems, he became increasingly anxious. His family reported worsening memory problems. A torn meniscus in the right knee and macular degeneration exacerbated his problems. Unable to take daily walks, he spent more time sitting at home. He stopped playing bridge with friends because of difficulty remembering and keeping track of the cards. Marvin became withdrawn, waking up confused, and cognitively impaired, often answering even simple questions with "I don't know."

9.2.4.2 Diagnosis and Treatment Plan

Seeking holistic treatment for the cognitive impairment, Marvin's family brought him for a neuropsychiatric consultation with an integrative psychiatrist. Marvin summed up his problems in the first evaluation session, "My family worries about my memory problems, but my real name is Worry." The differential diagnosis, which was discussed with Marvin and his family, included early dementia or possibly anxious depression, which can present as cognitive impairment, particularly in elderly patients. Marvin's family, among whom were two medical doctors, were anxious to get him worked up for dementia, and took him to a neurologist who found "slight age-related microvascular ischemia" on magnetic resonance imaging (MRI) and diagnosed mild cognitive impairment (MCI) but recommended no treatment. At this point, the etiology of the cognitive disorder was unclear.

The integrative psychiatrist discussed two treatment approaches with the family:

1. Cognitive enhancers with few side effects, including centrophenoxine (Meclofenoxate, Lucidril) and picamilon (a cerebral vasodilator) [21]. Picamilon, a cerebral vasodilator, is a composite of GABA and niacin (vitamin B3). Centrophenoxine is comprised of dimethyl-aminoethanol, a component in choline synthesis, and p-chlorophenoxyacetic acid, a synthetic plant growth hormone. It elevates brain acetylcholine, avidly scavenges free radicals, enhances antioxidants, and has shown some benefits for memory and cognitive function when combined with other nutrients and nootropics [22].
2. A Chinese herbal preparation, Free and Easy Wanderer Plus (FEWP) (by Golden Flower), which contained herbs used for anxiety, depression, weakness, and memory and cognitive decline.

In treating a geriatric patient, it is safest to start with the mildest agents in order to avoid potential side effects. Elderly patients are particularly susceptible, when given sedatives, anxiolytics, antidepressants, and other psychotropics, to experience sedation, somnolence, confusion, cognitive impairment, postural hypotension, syncope (fainting), loss of balance, falls resulting in fractures, incoordination, slurred speech, dyskinesias (repetitive involuntary movements), cardiac arrhythmias, gastrointestinal problems, and other serious side effects [23]. It would have been a mistake to give this patient a prescription anxiolytic such as clonazepam or alprazolam, because he would have been at risk particularly for confusion, worsening of depression, and possibly disinhibition of behavior [24].

Although the family tended to focus on the patient's cognitive problems, the patient himself had identified worry (anxiety) as the main issue. Even though this patient did not have dramatic outward signs of anxiety, the physician knew that it was important to listen to his identified complaint. Therefore, the provisional assessment was anxiety with cognitive/memory impairment and secondary depression. The old term "anxious depression" aptly described this presentation. Although anxiety disorders and mood disorders have been separated in the Diagnostic and Statistical Manual, Fifth Edition[DSM-5; 25], they are often comorbid, as in this patient. Free and Easy Wanderer Plus was chosen as the first treatment trial in order to address the patient's anxiety, depression, and mild cognitive impairment. Furthermore, elderly patients, who are often weak and frail, may benefit from the strengthening or "tonic" effects of these herbs [26].

Free and Easy Wanderer Plus (FEWP) is a 3000-year-old Chinese herbal formula comprised of 11 herbs: *Bupleurum chinense*, *Atractylodes macrocephalae*, *Poriacocus*, *Angelica sinensis*, *Lilium brownii*, *Rehmannia glutinosa*, *Paeonia lactiflora*, *Salvia miltiorrhiza*, *Mentha haplocalyx*, *Glycyrrhiza uralensis*, and *Zingiber officinale*. This formula has been studied in14 modern controlled trials in bipolar depression and poststroke depression, as an adjunct to conventional antidepressants, and for reduction of carbamazepine side effects [26, 27]. Grown in Taiwan, FEWP by Golden Flower is manufactured to British Herbal Pharmacopoeia standards with no contaminants. Six of the component herbs have calming, sedative, or anti-anxiety effects; two are mild antidepressants; four enhance memory or cognitive function; five have antifatigue and tonic effects; six have anti-inflammatory or antioxidant effects, or relieve joint pain (see Table 9.1). In clinical studies and in the author's (RPB) experience, about 50 % of patients have obvious improvement by 14 days. It requires a prescription from a medical physician or a certified herbalist in the United States. FEWP can be obtained with a prescription through websites, for example, www.DandelionBotanical.com.

9.2.4.3 Treatment outcome

After taking FEWP for 2 weeks, Marvin and his daughter reported that he was feeling much better. His worrying had stopped. Energy, interest, and motivation returned to his normal level. His memory improved such that he was able to resume his usual activities, socialize, and play bridge with friends.

9.2.4.4 Discussion

While it is challenging to decipher which of the constituents had the greatest effects on the patient, we could reasonably assume that the primary effects were calming, anxiolytic, and antidepressant. Secondary benefits, including memory and cognitive enhancement, could be attributed to improved cerebral circulation (vasodilation and antiplatelet action) and reduced inflammation and oxidative damage [28].

Like so many elderly patients, Marvin's life was in danger of becoming constricted by the anxiety, loss of interest and motivation, withdrawal, isolation, inactivity, and lack of stimulation that too often accelerate the decline into terminal states of physical and mental illness. We have much to learn about the mechanisms of action of herbal formulas, but we can still utilize them to help our patients, particularly those who are at risk for adverse events from conventional Western pharmaceuticals. Whether prescribing pharmaceutical medications or phytomedicines, observing and listening carefully to the patient, tuning into the patient's experience of the world through their disorder, and seeing past the most obvious symptoms are essential for correct diagnosis and effective treatment.

Table 9.1 Free and easy wanderer plus formulation

Latin name[a]	Pin Yin[b]	Common name	%[c]	Constituent[d]	mg/tab[e]	Effects partial list
Bupleurum chinense DC	RenShen (Hong)	Bupleurum Dry root	7.3	Saikosaponin	0.7	Depression, anxiety, fatigue, concentration, memory, physical endurance
Zingiber officinale	Sheng Jiang	Ginger (Fresh)	4.9			Calming
Atractylodes macrocephalae	Bai Zhu	Atractylodes (Alba) Dry root, stem	7.3	Atractylenolide	0.17	Joint pain
Angelica sinensis (Oliv) Diels	Dang gui	Chinese angelica Dry root	9.8	Ferulic acid	0.03	Blood pressure, joint pain, anemia
Poria cocos	Fu Shen	Poria Mushroom	7.3			Memory, anxiety, nervousness, fatigue
Lilium brownii	Bai he	Hong Kong lilly Squamous bulb	24.3			Sedative, tonic
Rehmannia glutinosa	Di-huang	Chinese foxglove Dry root	12.2	Catapol	4.4	Anti-inflammatory, stress, adrenal support, tonic
Paeonia lactiflora Pall	Bai Shao	Chinese peony Peeled dry root	9.8	Paeoniflorin	1.2	Anti-inflammatory, fatigue
Glycyrrhiza uralensis Fisch	Zhi Gan Cao	Licorice Dry root	2.4	Glycyrrhizic acid	0.6	Anti-inflammatory
Salvia miltiorrhiza	Dan-shen	Red sage Dry root	9.8	Tanshinone salvianolic	31.5 15.6	Stroke, ischemia, cerebral vasodilator, ↓platelet aggregation
Latin Name[a]	Pin Yin[b]	Common Name	%[c]	Constituent[d]	mg/tab[e]	Effects Partial List[6]
Polygala tenuifolia	Yuan Zhi	Polygala	11.8			Memory, cognition, antidepressant

Zingiber officinale	Sheng Jiang	Ginger Fresh root	4.9			calming
Mentha haplocalyx Briq	Bo he	Japanese peppermint Dry stem, dry leaf	4.9			Anti-inflammatory, antioxidant

Adapted from Li et al. [26]

Key: [a]FEWP formulas may vary among different producers.

[b]Each herb has numerous names in TCM and other Asian Medicines; 2 % proportion of each constituent within the total formulation.

[c]Some standardization constituents were not measured.

[d]Amount in mg not available for some constituents.

[e]Each herb has more effects and clinical uses than shown. This partial list shows only the effects relevant to Case#4

Conclusion

Anxiety can be overshadowed by a host of other symptoms, as illustrated in these four complex cases. Striking physical symptoms, such as dystonias, temporomandibular pain, headaches, functional bowel disorders, and chest pain, can become the focus of medical attention. When this occurs, the underlying anxiety that may be driving the physical condition may escape notice. A superficially successful life may conceal a traumatic past. The "treatment-resistant" patient (i.e. who does not respond well to conventional medications) may have drug sensitivities that require the combined use of mild herbal medicines. Patients with developmental disorders, learning disabilities, and communication impairments are particularly challenging. The urgent need for behavioral control often leads to the overuse of major tranquilizers that temporarily sedate the patient, miss the real target symptoms, and exacerbate underlying cognitive dysfunctions. Combining mild herbal, nutrient, and nootropic agents can alleviate anxiety and agitation, while improving verbal and cognitive functions enough to bring the patient to a higher level of functioning and quality of life. Distinguishing between the effects of anxiety/depression and cognitive dysfunction in geriatric patients is critical for treatment. What may appear to be an inexorable slide into dementia can often be halted by providing gentle, tolerable herbs and nutrients to relieve the less obvious emotional components while supporting optimal cognitive and social functioning.

References

1. Jellin PG, Gregory PJ. Pharmacist's letter/prescriber's letter natural medicines comprehensive database. 12th ed. Therapeutic Research: Stockton; 2009.
2. White DJ et al. Anti-stress, behavioural and magnetoencephalography effects of an l-theanine-based nutrient drink: a randomised, double-blind, placebo-controlled, crossover trial. Nutrients. 2016;8(1):53–72.
3. Lardner AL. Neurobiological effects of the green tea constituent theanine and its potential role in the treatment of psychiatric and neurodegenerative disorders. Nutr Neurosci. 2014;17(4):145–55.
4. Kirsch DL, Nichols F. Cranial electrotherapy stimulation for treatment of anxiety, depression, and insomnia. In: Muskin PR, Gerbarg PL, Brown RP editors. Complementary and Integrative Therapies for Psychiatric Disorders. Psych Clin NA. 2013;36(1):169–176.
5. Sageman S, Brown RP. 3-Acetyl-7-oxo-dehydroepiandrosterone for healing treatment-resistant posttraumatic stress disorder in women: 5 case reports [2]. J Clin Psychiatry. 2006;**67**(3):493–6.
6. Rasmusson AM et al. An increased capacity for adrenal DHEA release is associated with decreased avoidance and negative mood symptoms in women with PTSD. Neuropsychopharmacol. 2004;29(8):1546–57.
7. Mohamadpour AH et al. Safety evaluation of crocin (a constituent of saffron) tablets in healthy volunteers. Iran J Basic Med Sci. 2013;16(1):39–46.
8. Shahmansouri N et al. A randomized, double-blind, clinical trial comparing the efficacy and safety of Crocus sativus L. with fluoxetine for improving mild to moderate depression in post percutaneous coronary intervention patients. J Affect Disord. 2014;155(1):216–22.

9. Modabbernia A, Akhondzadeh S. Saffron, passionflower, valerian and sage for mental health. Psychiatr Clin N Am. 2013;36(1):85–91.
10. Pratte MA, Nanavati KB, Young V, Morley CP. An alternative treatment foranxiety: a systematic review of human trial results reported for the Ayurvedic herb ashwagandha (Withania somnifera). J Altern Complementary Med. 2014;20(12):901–8. doi: 10.1089/acm.2014.0177.
11. Delalleau B et al. Analysis of the side effects of tianeptine. Clin Neuropharmacol. 1988;11(Suppl 2):S83–9.
12. Atmaca M et al. Switching to tianeptine in patients with antidepressant-induced sexual dysfunction. Hum Psychopharmacol. 2003;18(4):277–80.
13. JA C e S. From restoration of neuroplasticity to the treatment of depression: clinical experience. Eur Neuropsychopharmacol. 2004;14(Suppl 5):S511–21.
14. Zoladz PR, Fleshner M, Diamond DM. Differential effectiveness of tianeptine, clonidine and amitriptyline in blocking traumatic memory expression, anxiety and hypertension in an animal model of PTSD. ProgNeuro-Psychopharmacol Biol Psychiatry. 2013;44:1–16.
15. Streeter CC et al. Effects of yoga on the autonomic nervous system, gamma-aminobutyric-acid, and allostasis in epilepsy, depression, and post-traumatic stress disorder. Med Hypotheses. 2012;78(5):571–9.
16. Abdou AM et al. Relaxation and immunity enhancement effects of gamma-aminobutyric acid(GABA) administration in humans. Biofactors. 2006;26(3):201–8.
17. Winblad B. Piracetam: a review of pharmacological properties and clinical uses. CNS Drug Rev. 2005;11(2):169–82.
18. Winnicka K, Tomasiak M, Bielawska A. Piracetaman old drug with novel properties? Acta Pol PharmDrug Res. 2005;62(5):405–9.
19. He Z et al. Piracetam ameliorated oxygen and glucose deprivation-induced injury in rat cortical neurons via inhibition of oxidative stress, excitatory amino acids release and P53/Bax. Cell Mol Neurobiol. 2014;34(4):539–47.
20. Graham KA et al. Double-blind, placebo-controlled investigation of amantadine for weight loss in subjects who gained weight with olanzapine. Am J Psychiatry. 2005;162(9):1744–6.
21. Brown RP, Gerbarg PL. Complementary and integrative treatments in brain injury. In: Silver JM, McAllister TW, Yudofsky SC, editors. Textbook of traumatic brain injury. 2 ed. Washington, DC: American Psychiatric Press, Inc.; 2011. p. 599–622.
22. Gerbarg PL, Brown RP. Phytomedicines for prevention and treatment of mental health disorders. Psychiatric Clin N Am. 2013;36(1):37–47.
23. Van Strien AM et al. Psychotropic medications, including short acting benzodiazepines, strongly increase the frequency of falls in elderly. Maturitas. 2013;74(4):357–62.
24. Gustafsson M et al. Association between behavioral and psychological symptoms and psychotropic drug use among old people with cognitive impairment living in geriatric care settings. Int Psychogeriatrics. 2013;25(9):1415–23.
25. American Psychiatric Association. Diagnostic and statistical manual of mental disorders. 5. ed. Arlington: American Psychiatric Association; 2013.
26. Li LT et al. The beneficial effects of the herbal medicine free and easy wanderer plus (FEWP) and fluoxetine on post-stroke depression. J Altern Complement Med. 2008;14(7):841–6.
27. Qin F et al. Meta-analysis of randomized controlled trials to assess the effectiveness and safety of free and easy wanderer plus, a polyherbal preparation for depressive disorders. JPsychiatr Res. 2011;45(11):1518–24.
28. Wang HN et al. Free and Easy Wanderer Plus (FEWP), a polyherbal preparation, ameliorates PTSD-like behavior and cognitive impairments in stressed rats. Prog Neuro-Psychopharmacol Biol Psychiatry. 2009;33(8):1458–63.

SAMe in the Treatment of Refractory Depression with Comorbid Anxiety: A Case Study in a High Histamine Patient

10

Rachel Arthur

10.1 Introduction

Imogen presented with treatment refractory depression; however, the most striking feature of her presentation and her most pressing concern was severe anxiety. This is a case in which a whole-system naturopathic approach was not initially used (e.g. treating every potential contributing system, such as digestion and sex hormones). Instead, due to the severity of her mental health issues, initial treatment was focused on neurotransmitter support. This case is a great illustration of how quickly, profoundly and sustainably complementary medicines can work in certain mental health cases, even cases as serious as this one.

10.2 Case Presentation

10.2.1 Presenting Complaint

Imogen was 61 years old and experiencing her fifth episode of major depression (based on her recollection). Her previous episodes were severe and included suicidal ideation and intent and had required extended voluntary hospitalisation on two occasions. In her 40s she experienced short-term efficacy with an SSRI (fluoxetine); however, subsequent trials during depressive episodes since had been unsuccessful. In addition, she had unsuccessfully trialled a long list of medications including other SSRIs, SNRIs, tricyclics, antipsychotics, mood stabilisers, and even electroconvulsive therapy (ECT). She reported consistent anxiolytic relief with benzodiazepines only.

R. Arthur
School of Health and Human Sciences, Southern Cross University,
Lismore, New South Wales, Australia
e-mail: rachel@rachelarthur.com.au

D. Camfield et al. (eds.), *Evidence-Based Herbal and Nutritional Treatments for Anxiety in Psychiatric Disorders*, DOI 10.1007/978-3-319-42307-4_10

Although her diagnosis of depression was not made until her early 40s, Imogen reports marked anxiety from childhood onwards. Being adopted, she attributed some of this to psychosocial factors; however, her recollection of anxious thoughts and behaviours were striking and pervasive. Imogen met her biological parents in her 20s and discovered that her father experienced anxiety and that two of his other children also had mental health diagnoses, one with bipolar II disorder and another with severe treatment refractory depression.

Imogen's current depressive episode began 2 months prior, during which time she had been under the care of a psychiatrist, psychologist (treated with cognitive–behaviour therapy), and general practitioner (GP). Over this period, she had again trialled several different psychiatric medications, each marred by poor tolerance and a lack of clinical improvement. At the time of presenting she was being weaned off a tricyclic (nortriptyline), due to the experience of marked anticholinergic side effects (i.e. blurred vision, low blood pressure and confusion), and her psychiatrist had advised her that her only remaining option was further ECT sessions. Her diagnosis was treatment refractory major depressive disorder with anxious distress.

Key symptoms at presentation included:

- Impaired sleep onset and maintenance
- Early morning waking with inability to resume sleep
- Waking with severe psychomotor agitation, including sweating, shaking, tachycardia, diarrhoea and racing thoughts
- Impaired appetite, greatly diminished self-care, weight loss of ≈3 kg over 2 months
- Hair loss

Due to poor mental health, Imogen had been unemployed for the past 3 years. She was single and had one adult child with cystic fibrosis who lived independently. Imogen had been taking hormone replacement therapy (HRT) for the past 11 years and had been advised by her GP to continue with this. She also reported a long history of irritable bowel syndrome (IBS)-C type symptoms including bloating, incomplete evacuation and flatulence, for which she routinely took an osmotic laxative. She was diagnosed with osteopenia (early stages of osteoporosis) in her late 50s.

10.2.2 Assessment of Patient

Imogen was unable to complete a baseline Depression Anxiety and Stress Scale (DASS) assessment due to the nortriptyline-induced confusion and presenting agitation. However, in the following month, her DASS scores placed her in the extremely severe category for the "Stress" subscale, in the moderate category for the "Anxiety" subscale, and the severe category for the "Depression" subscale.

She was normotensive (118/75 mmHg) and displayed orthostatic hypotension (likely the result of nortriptyline). Her post-prandial (2 h) blood glucose level was 5.2 mmol/L and urinalysis, which were all normal. Recent pathology results revealed: low plasma zinc at 9 μmol/L, an elevated 9 am cortisol at 545 nmol/L, healthy homocysteine at 6.5 mmol/L and evidence of suboptimal magnesium and potassium levels. Her blood histamine was 0.6 μmol/L. She had a long history of low positive C-reactive protein (CRP), fluctuating between 1 and 2 mg/L.

10.2.3 Diagnosis and Treatment Plan

Differential naturopathic diagnoses, supporting and counter-indications.

Differential naturopathic diagnoses	Supportive evidence	Counter-indications
Monoamine theory of depression, e.g. low serotonin	Presents with depression and anxiety	Lack of efficacy of SSRIs and TCAs
Neuro-inflammation	Long-term detectable CRP Elevated neutrophil counts since 2010	Lack of raised monocytes Lack of "sickness like behaviour" [1] Hx of elevated neutrophils could potentially be related to specific infections at the time rather than general inflammation
High histamine	Elevated blood histamine Clinical features consistent with this: Chronic anxious features Difficulty with relaxing, winding down, initiating sleep Highly motivated, good cognition Initial partial benefit from SSRIs GI bloating and diarrhoea [2]	No inhalant or seasonal allergies which are typical of high histamine cases
HPA over-activation	Marked anxiety with sweating, trembling, early morning waking, racing thoughts, tachycardia High morning cortisol Anxiety symptoms are worst in morning and tend to reduce by late afternoon Evidence of low magnesium and potassium which result from high cortisol due to increased renal losses	Unclear as to whether this is a cause or consequence
Low GABA	Anxiety features Efficacy of benzodiazepines	Unclear as to whether this is a cause or consequence
Zinc deficiency	Evidence of low plasma zinc since at least since 2009 Low zinc levels have been proposed as a marker of treatment-resistant depression [3] and several studies suggest a positive clinical effect using zinc as an adjunctive or stand-alone therapy [4]	

Note. CRP C-reactive protein, *GI* gastrointestinal

The naturopathic diagnosis was that Imogen's constitutional tendency to high histamine was the key underpinning driver behind her depression and anxiety. This was being compounded by a zinc deficiency and suboptimal magnesium and potassium levels, the latter two being secondary to the significant HPA activation that is characteristic of anxiety.

Initial lifestyle and behavioural recommendations included:

- Reduce or eliminate all sources of caffeine
- Try to eat regularly (e.g. every 4 h)
- Include a high-quality protein at every meal (e.g. tinned salmon with lunch)
- Increase fish consumption to 3/7 days
- Consume "smoothies" (high protein/fibre/antioxidant) for breakfast 3/7 days to address low appetite and improve overall nutrient density
- Consume one glass of vegetable juice every day to get around low appetite and improve overall nutrient density
- Maintain regular gentle, pleasurable, social, exercise with walking, yoga, and swimming

Following full washout of the last TCA, the initial prescription was stand-alone magnesium repletion and simple use of kava (*Piper methysticum)* as Mediherb tablets extract equivalent to dry root containing kava lactones 50 mg 3.2 g administered as two tablets up to three times a day; however, this was ineffective. Subsequently, the following interventions were recommended, which were introduced in a staggered fashion over approximately 1 month.

Intervention	Dose per Serve	Daily dosage regime	Brand	Rationale
Zinc	25 mg elemental	One capsule	Double strength zinc picolinate (Thorne)	Correction of zinc deficiency
Magnesium	175 mg elemental	One tablet BD	Organic magnesium (Thompsons)	Magnesium repletion in the context of ongoing excess HPA activity which can then help to reduce HPA activation [5]
Vitamin C	1 gm sustained release	One tablet BD	Sustained-release vitamin C (Blackmores)	Repletion of Vitamin C in context of ongoing excess HPA activity which can help to buffer the physiological impact of high cortisol [6] and has been shown to lower anxiety [7]
Theanine	200 mg	Two capsules on waking and pm	Theanine (Thorne)	GABAminergic effects either via a direct increase in GABA levels or via activity at the GABA receptors [8] *Specifically given for symptomatic relief of anxiety on waking*
SAMe	400 mg	One tablet BD (mane)	SAMe 400 (Nutrition care)	Support of histamine clearance ➔ anxiolytic and antidepressant [9, 10]

10.3 Treatment Outcome

Initial treatment outcomes were based on self-report during clinical interview. While the first prescription (high-dose magnesium and kava) was ineffective, administration of theanine prn produced significant fast-acting anxiolysis (within the hour). With the subsequent introduction of SAMe, Imogen reported longer-lasting relief from anxiety; within 2 weeks of initiation she said, "I feel like my whole system is starting to calm down," and reported absence of early morning waking with anxiety, and absence of diarrhoea and sweating, improved sleep quality and a reduced need for theanine.

Within a month, Imogen started to reduce her intake of supplements in response to significant mood improvements, taking the theanine only when waking instead of throughout the day and only one daily dose of SAMe. Within 6 weeks of her initial improvements, she began organising an overseas working trip, which she had regarded as untenable at the first appointment. Imogen maintained her reduced supplement regime while overseas for 3 months.

Since this time (3 years ago) Imogen has maintained more or less the same supplement regime with great success. Repeat DASS assessments, performed quarterly on average, suggest her depressive and anxious features are all within the "normal range." Updated pathology results reflect some improvements with her plasma zinc levels increased to 12 umol/L and resolution of low magnesium/potassium. Repeat cortisol levels also have fallen within range.

During this period, Imogen has returned to paid work, started a long-term relationship and moved home. She has also endured multiple stressors without relapse; however, when experiencing increased stress, she resumes taking the higher prescribed doses of SAMe and theanine as part of her management plan. She continues to see a psychologist for support when needed and maintains regular check-ups with both myself and her GP, but has not needed to see a psychiatrist for years.

10.4 Discussion

Naturopathic medicine does not always need to address all body systems to be effective. The intervention employed in this case was consistent with a holistic naturopathic approach that required a staged approach to treatment. The priority was to stabilise Imogen's mental health symptoms before addressing her long-standing digestive problems. While Imogen's mood improvements came relatively quickly, targeted interventions for her long-standing digestive symptoms did not start until at least 6–9 months into treatment, and following that specific attention was paid to improving her sex hormone imbalances. This case has been a useful reminder that it is necessary to focus treatment on a patient's more severe primary concerns before addressing secondary presentations.

This case is also a good example of a patient presenting with high histamine and mental health concerns. The treatment approach presented in this case study comes from the original research by Pfeiffer, who proposed that an imbalance in histamine (via accelerated or impaired degradation) could be a contributing factor to mental health conditions including depression and anxiety [11]. In addition to measurement of histamine or other related markers of methylation, Pfeiffer proposed a set of signs and symptoms believed to be attributable to the "high" or "low histamine" state, which assist identification. The high histamine, or "histadelic" individual, according to his theory, may present with "severe depression, easy crying, insomnia, obsessive compulsive ruminations, and suicidality" [9]. This underscores the role of histamine as an important excitatory neurotransmitter as well as an allergic mediator. Based on this hypothesis, treatment with SAMe as a critical co-factor for histamine degradation via the HMNT pathway is indicated and may help to correct this histadelia.

SAMe has evidence as an effective stand-alone and adjunctive antidepressant in a wide range of patients and presentations including some well-recognised complex co-morbidities such as Parkinson's disease [10]. To date, there is no evidence from clinical trials for the efficacy of SAMe as a treatment for anxiety symptoms, and histamine was not found to moderate the treatment response to SAMe in treating MMD [9]. However, clinical experience in successfully using SAMe in patients with depression, anxiety, dysthymia, and some eating disorders concurs with Pfeiffer's model of heterogeneous biochemistry amongst individuals who present with the "same diagnosis" and, specifically attests to a sub-population of individuals with high histamine and therefore more likely to achieve treatment effectiveness with this nutraceutical.

References

1. Maes M, Berk M, Goehler L, Song C, Anderson G, Galecki P, et al. Depression and sickness behavior are Janus-faced responses to shared inflammatory pathways. BMC Med. 2012;10:66.
2. Maintz L, Novak N. Histamine and histamine intolerance. Am J Clin Nutr. 2007;85(5):1185–96.
3. Siwek M, Szewczyk B, Dudek D, Styczen K, Sowa-Kucma M, Mlyniec K, et al. Zinc as a marker of affective disorders. Pharmacol Rep. 2013;65(6):1512–8.
4. Swardfager W, Herrmann N, McIntyre RS, Mazereeuw G, Goldberger K, Cha DS, et al. Potential roles of zinc in the pathophysiology and treatment of major depressive disorder. Neurosci Biobehav Rev. 2013;37(5):911–29.
5. Sartori SB, Whittle N, Hetzenauer A, Singewald N. Magnesium deficiency induces anxiety and HPA axis dysregulation: modulation by therapeutic drug treatment. Neuropharmacology. 2012;62(1):304–12.
6. Brody S, Preut R, Schommer K, Schurmeyer TH. A randomized controlled trial of high dose ascorbic acid for reduction of blood pressure, cortisol, and subjective responses to psychological stress. Psychopharmacology (Berl). 2002;159(3):319–24.
7. de Oliveira IJ, de Souza VV, Motta V, Da-Silva SL. Effects of oral vitamin C supplementation on anxiety in students: adouble-blind, randomized, placebo-controlled trial. Pak J Biol Sci. 2015;18(1):11–8.
8. Nathan PJ, Lu K, Gray M, Oliver C. The neuropharmacology of L-theanine(N-ethyl-L-glutamine): a possible neuroprotective and cognitive enhancing agent. J Herb Pharmacother. 2006;6(2):21–30.
9. Sarris J, Papakostas GI, Vitolo O, Fava M, Mischoulon D. S-adenosyl methionine (SAMe) versus escitalopram and placebo in major depression RCT: efficacy and effects of histamine and carnitine as moderators of response. J Affect Disord. 2014;164:76–81.

10. Papakostas GI, Mischoulon D, Shyu I, Alpert JE, Fava M. S-adenosyl methionine (SAMe) augmentation of serotonin reuptake inhibitors for antidepressant nonresponders with major depressive disorder: a double-blind, randomized clinical trial. Am J Psychiatry. 2010;167(8):942–8.
11. Pfeiffer CC. Nutrition and mental illness: an orthomolecular approach tobalancing body chemistry. Rochester: Healing Art Press; 1988.

A Complex Case of Undiagnosed Generalised Anxiety Disorder with Episodic Panic Attacks

11

Jane Hutchens

11.1 Introduction

This case study explores the assessment and management of generalised anxiety disorder (GAD) and has been chosen due to the unique diagnostic challenges, multiple drug allergies and potential drug interactions that characterised the case, as well as the broader impact the client's diagnosis of GAD on her family.

11.2 Case Presentation

11.2.1 Presenting Complaint

Debra first presented when she was 53 years old and was seeking support to manage her bone density, facilitate weight loss, and to optimise her health following a diagnosis of breast cancer 10 months prior. Debra had a lumpectomy and removal of several axillary lymph nodes followed by 30 sessions of external beam radiation. Recent bone mineral density assessment identified osteopaenia in the neck of the femur and osteoporosis in the lumbar spine.

Previous history included an old back strain following a fall and pneumonia 12 months prior. She has known allergies to Sulphur, Penicillin, Roxithyromycin (Rulide) in addition to marked side effects (nausea and vomiting) from codeine, and hot sweats from rhubarb. In addition, Debra reported a poorly defined reaction to vitamin C supplements in which she experienced altered taste and mouth numbness; it is not clear if the reaction was to an excipient or the form of vitamin C, colouring or some other factor; she is able to tolerate vitamin C rich foods.

J. Hutchens
Lemongrove Road Holistic Health, Penrith, NSW, Australia
e-mail: janehutchens@hotmail.com

D. Camfield et al. (eds.), *Evidence-Based Herbal and Nutritional Treatments for Anxiety in Psychiatric Disorders*, DOI 10.1007/978-3-319-42307-4_11

Debra is married and has three adult children, all of who were living at home. She works full-time in a residential facility for people living with disabilities. Her family history included significant allergies in both of her siblings, parents, and one grandparent. In addition, her father had died from lung cancer and had multiple sclerosis. Her father and two siblings had been diagnosed and treated for depression.

11.3 Assessment of Patient

11.3.1 Initial Assessment

Debra did not present initially for mental health concerns and no overt features of anxiety were observed as defined by the DSM-V [1]. During the case history, she disclosed experiencing depression following her diagnosis of cancer and having sought support from a psychologist at the cancer centre she attended, and that she felt that was a constructive and positive experience. Debra stated that she no longer felt depressed and denied any other mental health concerns during the initial consultation. Thus, the original assessments related to the reason she sought a consultation and included basic biochemical and metabolic assessments.

Over the following 12 months, Debra reported persistently elevated levels of stress, with triggers at work, in her marriage, her upcoming annual cancer check, and family health concerns. During this time she felt that physical exercise and some basic cognitive re-framing exercises were sufficient in managing her stress. Herbal anxiolytics were suggested and declined, as was the suggestion that counselling may be helpful. She reported that to some extent she "thrives" on the intensity of the type of work she does, and has never been a person to "lay around reading all day." At this time she was still sleeping well, able to perform her job to the same standards, and had not altered social or family activity due to the stress.

11.3.2 Ongoing Assessment

Fourteen months after the initial consultation, Debra experienced a further, and significant, escalation of her stress as a result of serious family health concerns, children undergoing difficult times, financial strain and a prolonged episode of bronchitis.The following month she felt that her overall level of stress had decreased, though work was beginning to intensify due to annual additional workload requirements.

Two years and 3 months after the initial presentation, Debra reported feeling "tingling" in her feet and lower legs, and that they "felt puffy." At times this extended to her arms and face as well. She had experienced tingling and swelling in response to sulphur drugs and penicillin. On a couple of occasions she had an unusual taste in her mouth that was not dissimilar to what she experienced with vitamin C supplements. There were no changes to any aspect of her life prior to these sensations and generally feels well other than being concerned about the paraesthesias due to her family history of MS. The first episode occurred on the way home from holidays, where she did not alter diet, supplements or medications. Debra was concerned and puzzled but not distressed by these symptoms.

Assessment by her oncologist included ceasing all medication to exclude them as being causative, a bilateral lower-limb Doppler's ultrasound to exclude deep venous thrombosis, full-body CT scan, biochemistry assessment and physical examination. Nil abnormalities were identified. Assessment by a neurologist (seeking to exclude MS) identified nil abnormalities.

Upon reviewing the results, Debra's general practitioner (GP) suggested she was experiencing anxiety. A broader exploration of her history revealed two second-degree relatives with bipolar disorder, that one sibling likely had significant anxiety as well as the previously mentioned depression, three of her sibling's children had behavioural/neurological disorders, her mother likely had undiagnosed GAD with significant behavioural effects, and one of her daughters likely had an undiagnosed GAD. Later discussion revealed that another daughter had quite rigid thinking and a tendency to perfectionism, possibly with underlying anxiety.

11.3.3 Diagnosis and Treatment Plan

Debra returned for a consultation once the GP had assessed the symptoms to be those of anxiety. She was referred to a clinical psychologist whom she saw regularly for several months and who assessed her as having a GAD with episodic panic attacks. In the following year, Debra reflected on her life and health and was able to identify numerous occasions spanning at least 30 years that were likely to be mild panic attacks.

11.3.4 Therapeutics Goals

The new therapeutics goals for Debra included:

1. Reduce symptoms of anxiety
2. Reduce or eliminate panic attacks
3. Further develop behavioural strategies to reduce stress and anxiety
4. Ensure appropriate diet
5. Support adrenal and nervous systems function
6. Reduce recurrence or severity of recurrence of anxiety and panic attacks

11.3.5 Prescribed Treatment

The treatment plan built on existing exercise, relaxation and nutritional plans.

1. *Exercise*: Debra exercised at least 4 times a week, a combination of cardio and resistance.

2. *Relaxation techniques*: These were primarily reinforcing techniques prescribed by the psychologist and included breathing techniques, progressive relaxation and guided meditation.
3. *Nutrition*: Her diet already included omega 3 fatty acids, a wide range of vegetables, good levels of hydration, adequate protein and little caffeine, sugar or alcohol.
4. *Nutritional Supplementation*: Magnesium 300 mg before bed was added to the supplements Debra was already taking (calcium, vitamin D and Omega 3 fatty acids).
5. *Bodywork*: Continued monthly oncology massage and chiropractic interventions.
6. *Herbal medicine*: Debra had difficulty tolerating liquid herbs thus the following tablet formulation was used:

   Anxioton by bioconcepts
   Per tablet
   Melissa officinalis (Lemon Balm) dry leaf and flowers 750 mg
   Passiflora incarnata (Passionflower) dry herb top flowering 1.5 g
   Piper methysticum (Kava Kava) dry root extract 4 g, Kavalactones 40 mg
   Magnolia officinalis (Magnolia) dry stem bark 1.5 g
   Zizyphus jujuba (Zizyphus) dry seed extract 3 g
   Glycine100 mg
   Magnesium amino acid chelate 100 mg, equivalent to Magnesium 50 mg
   Dose: two to four tablets orally per day

11.4 Treatment Outcome

Debra underwent a thorough physical assessment but did not complete any validated psychometric assessments; assessment was based on clinical interview and self-reported symptoms.

The first follow-up after commencement of Anxioton was planned for 1 month but did not occur until 2 months due to Christmas break and Debra feeling improved and not seeking a consultation sooner. At this visit she reported feeling "really good" on the Anxioton. She had fewer panic episodes and those she had she felt able to "breathe through" and prevent from escalating. Due to her history of drug allergies and sensitivities, she started with one tablet per day to assess any reaction, then once confident she increased gradually to 1 morning and 2 at night. Debra was able to titrate her dose effectively according to her symptoms.

Debra began seeing the psychologist in another 2 months' time (4 months after commencing the Anxioton). She described the counselling sessions as helpful and in particular they were useful in exploring her family history and dynamics. In addition to the new techniques learnt for managing anxiety, Debra was able to introduce the issue of anxiety with several family members and as a result two family members subsequently sought professional help for their anxiety with good effect.

Debra continued the Anxioton, counselling, nutritional and lifestyle strategies in the following 14 months. She initially maintained the Anxioton dose of 3 per day, then after 6 months reduced the dose to one mane, as that was how it was most beneficial for her. After another 3 months she took herself off the Anxioton, though maintained a supply should she require some.

In this time Debra has experienced significant stressors with family ill-health, all of her children moving out of home, becoming a grandparent, one child moving overseas, relationship stressors with her birth family, inordinate demands in the workplace, an extended period of chest infection and antibiotic use, minor surgery, conflict between her surgeon and oncologist about treatment approaches and the marriage of one child. Debra adhered to all of the strategies above and had no panic attacks, could recognise escalating stress and was able to self-manage effectively. Indeed, she felt a sense of accomplishment and pride that she able to manage during such challenging times.

In addition to the improvement in her anxiety, during the treatment period Debra lost 17 kg of weight and reduced her body fat to within the healthy range, normalised her abnormal lipid profile and had a slight improvement in her neck of femur bone density. Her checks for breast cancer remain negative and she describes feeling better than she ever has.

11.5 Discussion

It was imperative to employ a simple approach in supporting Debra due to previous drug reactions and side effects, as well as the desire to not add to her stress by recommending a complicated and demanding treatment regime. In addition, Debra had received a strongly expressed negative opinion and advice about herbal medicine and nutritional supplements from her oncologist, and it was important to not create conflict and further angst by opposing this advice too dramatically.

Debra's diet was balanced and she had healthy digestive function, which increased the likelihood that she consumed and absorbed nutrients adequately. A variety of protein sources as well as adequate intake of approximately 70/g per day is likely to have provided the necessary amino acids required for the production of neurotransmitters.

Magnesium was added due to Debra experiencing some muscle cramps in her feet and for its role in neurological function. Magnesium has been shown to reduce hippocampal kindling, reduce the release of adrenocorticotrophic hormone (ACTH) and affect adrenocortical sensitivity to ACTH, which is amplified in stress [2–5]. It is suggested that where calcium and glutamate are excitatory and activate the *N*-methyl-d-aspartate (NMDA) receptor, that magnesium dampens NMDA activity and is thus inhibitory. γ-Aminobutyric acid is the central inhibitory neurotransmitter and magnesium interacts with the benzodiazepine/GABA-α receptors to elicit an anxiolytic effect [2, 3].

Omega 3 fatty acids have relatively little research in their application for anxiety, though some evidence exists that lower levels are associated with depression and anxiety[6] and that supplementation and/or dietary sources may reduce the incidence of anxiety and ameliorate symptoms [7, 8].

The herbal medicines in the Anxioton tablet were *Melissa officinalis*, *Passiflora incarnate*, *Piper methysticum, Magnolia officinalis and Zizyphus jujube,* all of which exhibited GABA-α receptor inhibition, which accounts for the empirical understanding of these herbs as anxiolytics and hypnotics [9].

11.5.1 Reflection

Debra's primary mental health carer was her psychologist; however, it would have been useful as her naturopath to conduct some quantitative measure of her anxiety that could be repeated at future consultations. Being able to perform objective, quantifiable assessments is essential in monitoring and evaluating treatment efficacy, thus enabling modification of approach, and it is perhaps especially important in mental health conditions where there is typically an absence of biochemical or other assessment measures, and where the subjective experience may be more difficult to analyse and determine. Simple tools such as the Depression and Anxiety Scale (DASS) [10], or a quality of life measure such as the validated Quality of Life Scale [11], or the Measure Yourself Medical Outcome Profile (MYMOP2) Questionnaire [12], which is a patient-centred outcome measure that can be applied to any clinical presentation could have been instructive.

This case highlights the need to commence each repeat consultation with a double focus; resuming the therapeutic conversation and re-evaluating information from previous consultations as well as being vigilant in observing and analysing without the encumbrance of presumed knowledge of the client. Upon the presentation of new symptomatology, it is essential to revisit the original client history documented and see if there are any clues that may be useful; in this case, the family history of mental health conditions warranted further exploration earlier than was undertaken. Finally, this case also demonstrates that a targeted and simple treatment approach can be very effective and without side effects.

References

1. American Psychiatric Association. Diagnostic and statistical manual of mental disorders: DSM-5. 5 ed. Washington, DC: American Psychiatric Association; 2013.
2. Murck H. Magnesium and affective disorders. Nutr Neurosci. 2002;5(6):375–89.
3. Poleszak E. Benzodiazepine/GABA(A) receptors are involved in magnesium-induced anxiolytic-like behavior in mice. Pharmacol Rep. 2008;60(4):483–9.
4. Poleszak E, Wlaz P, Wróbel A, Fidecka S, Nowak G. NMDA/glutamate mechanism of magnesium-induced anxiolytic-like behavior in mice. Pharmacol Rep. 2008;60(5):655–63.
5. Abumaria N, Yin B, Zhang L, Li X-Y, Chen T, Descalzi G, Zhao L, Ahn M, Luo L, Ran C, Zhuo M, Liu G. Effects of elevation of brain magnesium on fear conditioning, fear extinction, and synaptic plasticity in the infralimbic prefrontal cortex and lateral amygdala. J Neurosci. 2011;31(42):14871–81.

6. Lui J, Galfalvy H, Cooper T, Oquendo M, Grunebaum M, Mann J, Sublette M. Omega-3 polyunsaturated fatty acid status in major depression with comorbid anxiety disorders. J Clin Psychiatry. 2013;74(7):732–8.
7. Buydens-Branchey L, Branchey M, Hibbeln JR. Associations between increases in plasma n-3 polyunsaturated fatty acids following supplementation and decreases in anger and anxiety in substance abusers. Prog Neuropsychopharmacol Biol Psychiatry. 2008;32:568–75.
8. Kiecolt-Glaser JK, Belury MA, Andridge R, Malarkey WB, Glaser R. Omega-3 supplementation lowers inflammation and anxiety in medical students: a randomized controlled trial. Brain Behav Immun. 2011;25:1725–34.
9. Sarris J, McIntyre E, Camfield D. Plant-based medicines for anxiety disorders, part 2: areview of clinical studies with supporting preclinical evidence. CNS Drugs. 2013;27(4):301–19.
10. Lovibond SH, Lovibond PF. Manual for the depression anxiety stress scales. 2 ed. Sydney: Psychology Foundation; 1995.
11. Burckhardt C, Anderson K. The Quality of Life Scale (QOLS): reliability, validity, and utilization. Health Qual Life Outcomes. 2003;1:60.
12. Paterson C. Patient-centred outcome measurement. In: Macpherson H, Hammerschlag R, Lewith G, Schnyer R, editors. Acupuncture research: strategies for establishing an evidence base. London: Churchill Livingstone; 2007.

Herb and Nutrient-Drug Interaction Table

This table provides an overview of the drugs that have been found to interact with the herbal and nutritional medicines discussed in this book. The table is intended to be used as a quick reference guide only and is not exhaustive. As always, due diligence is required on a case-by-case basis when making clinical judgements. If a class of drug is not listed here, there was no known interaction found during literature search at the time of publication. However, for many of the herbal extracts listed in the table, further research is required in order to properly establish (or rule out) evidence for herb-drug interactions. The table is organised by drug class. The level of interaction is indicated using the following key:

- *SI* = Serious interaction
- *UC* = Use caution
- *OB* = Clinical observation needed
- *BI* = Potential beneficial interaction
- *CYP* = Cytochrome P450

D. Camfield et al. (eds.), *Evidence-Based Herbal and Nutritional Treatments for Anxiety in Psychiatric Disorders*, DOI 10.1007/978-3-319-42307-4

Drug class	Herb	Potential interaction	Evidence	Recommendations
Alcohol				
	Piper methysticum	*SI* = additive effect	Kava has a synergic effect with CNS depressants [1]	Avoid combining with alcohol [1]. Observe in patients who consume moderate to high amounts of alcohol
	Schisandra chinensis	*BI* = decreased side effects	Theoretically based on pharmacological action. In vivo study demonstrated hepatoprotective effects in induced liver damage [2]	Possible beneficial interaction
	Silybum marianum	*BI* = decreased side effects	Several studies demonstrating hepatoprotective effect of St Mary's thistle indicate this herb may reduce hepatic tissue damage related to alcohol consumption [3, 4]	Possible beneficial interaction
	N-Acetylcysteine	*BI* = decreased side effects	Evidence to suggest that NAC promotes the metabolism of alcohol and decreases damage to the liver and heart [5, 6]	Beneficial interaction
Anaesthetics (general)				
	Hypericum perforatum (St. John's wort)	*SI* = reduced drug effectiveness	Known interaction with CYP enzymes [7]	Avoid concurrent use. Discontinue 2–3 weeks prior to surgery [8]
Analgesics				
Codeine	*Piper methysticum*	*UC* = additive effect	Kava has a synergic effect with CNS depressants [1]	Medical supervision and monitoring of patient advised
Morphine	*Piper methysticum*	*UC* = additive effect	Kava has a synergic effect with CNS depressants [1]	Medical supervision and monitoring of patient advised
	Withania somnifera	*BI* = decreased drug tolerance and dependence	In vivo studies demonstrated inhibited morphine tolerance and dependence [9]. Efficacy not yet demonstrated in clinical trials	Possible beneficial interaction

Paracetamol	*Schisandra chinensis*	*BI*=decreased side effects	Based on pharmacological action, may have a hepatoprotective effect against liver damage from paracetamol [3, 4]	Possible beneficial interaction
	Silybum marianum	*BI*=decreased side effects	Based on pharmacological action, may have a hepatoprotective effect against liver damage from paracetamol [3]	Possible beneficial interaction
	N-Acetylcysteine	*BI*=decreased side effects	NAC is a proven antidote for acetaminophen overdose, as reviewed in a study of over 2540 patients. Most protective when NAC is taken within 8 h of paracetamol ingestion [10]	Beneficial interaction as well as being a treatment for paracetamol overdose (typically administered intravenously in a hospital setting in the case of overdose)
Anticonvulsants				
Anticonvulsants (general)	*Ginkgo biloba*	*UC*=reduced drug effectiveness	One case report of fatal seizure. Possible interaction with valproic acid and phenytoin, reducing drug effectiveness [8]	Observe patient with concurrent use. Interaction risk is low for standardized extracts at doses of 240 mg/day or lower [11]
	Hypericum perforatum	*SI*=reduced drug effectiveness	Known interaction with CYP enzymes effecting drug metabolism. May cause decreased drug effectiveness [7]	Avoid concurrent use
Carbamazepine	*Hypericum perforatum*	*OB*=possible reduced drug effectiveness	Induction of CYP enzymes, with potential increased drug metabolism; however, it has been reported not to have an effect on carbamazepine kinetics [12]	Observe patient with concurrent use; however, interaction is unlikely [8]
Phenobarbitone	*Piper methysticum*	*UC*=additive sedative effects	Demonstrated anticonvulsant activity [13]	Unknown clinical significance
Phenobarbitone and phenytoin	*Piper methysticum*	*UC*=additive sedative effects	In vitro seizure models demonstrated anticonvulsant activity [13]	Unknown clinical significance
	Hypericum perforatum	*UC*=reduced drug effectiveness	Induction of CYP enzymes, with potentially increased drug metabolism; however, it has not been reported in clinical studies [7]	Observe patient with concurrent use; however, interaction is unlikely [8]

(continued)

(continued)

Drug class	Herb	Potential interaction	Evidence	Recommendations
Antidepressants				
Atypical (bupropion)	*Hypericum perforatum*	*SI* = additive effect	Concurrent use may increase serotonin reuptake inhibition [7]	Avoid concurrent use, unless under medical supervision. Potential for serotonin syndrome with concurrent use. Use low-hyperforin extracts such as Ze117 [12]
Selective serotonin reuptake inhibitors and serotonin and norepinephrine reuptake inhibitors	*Ginkgo biloba*	*BO* = potential additive effects	A case report in a patient with Alzheimer's disease suggested a possible increase in the function of GABA receptors leading to sedation with concurrent use of trazodone [32]. However, clinically significant interactions appear to be dose dependent [11]	Observe patient with concurrent use. Interaction risk is low for standardized extracts at doses of 240 mg/day or lower [11]
	Hypericum perforatum	*SI* = additive effect	Induces CYP enzymes and P-glycoprotein. Pharmacokinetic trials and case studies reporting symptoms of serotonin syndrome [7, 8, 14]	Avoid concurrent use, unless under medical supervision. Potential for serotonergic syndrome with concurrent use. Use low-hyperforin extract such as Ze117 [12]
	Myo-inositol	*OB* = potential additive effects (although unconfirmed)	Due to the theories of serotonergic mechanism of action of MI, caution should be exercised when using in conjunction with antidepressants or St. John's wort. However, no reported cases of serotonin syndrome associated with MI to date [15]	Observe patient due to possible additive effects/hypomanic state
	Piper methysticum	*UC* = additive effect	Case study (combination valerian and kava preparation) increased lethargy when combined with paroxetine [8]	Mechanism of interaction unknown. Observe patient with concurrent use

Tricyclics	*Hypericum perforatum*	*SI* = reduced drug effectiveness	May decrease plasma levels of tricyclics and increase serotonin [12]	Avoid concurrent use, unless under medical supervision. Potential for serotonergic syndrome with concurrent use. Use low-hyperforin extracts such as Ze117 [12]
Ginkgo biloba	*Silybum marianum*	*BI* = reduced drug side effects	Based on pharmacological action, may have a hepatoprotective effect against drug-induced liver damage [3]	Possible beneficial interaction
Antihistamines				
Fexofenadine	*Hypericum perforatum*	*UC* = reduced drug effectiveness	Pharmacokinetic trials demonstrating decreased blood concentration of fexofenadine with concurrent use [8]	Avoid concurrent use to ensure treatment effectiveness
Antipsychotics				
Haloperidol	*Ginkgo biloba*	*OB* = additive effect and reduced side effects	Clinical trial demonstrating increased effects with concurrent use and decreased extrapyramidal side effects [16]	Mechanism of interaction unconfirmed. Observe patient and exercise caution with concurrent use. Interaction risk is low for standardized extracts at doses of 240 mg/day or lower [11]
Risperidone	*Ginkgo biloba*	*OB* = additive effect	Case study reporting priapism, possibly due to vasodilation effects [6]. One clinical trial reported no significant side effects with concurrent treatment [11]. EGb 761 (standardized *Ginkgo biloba* extract) has not demonstrated interaction effects in clinical trials [6]	Mechanism of interaction unconfirmed. Observe patient and use caution with concurrent use. Interaction risk is low for standardized extracts at doses of 240 mg/day or lower [11]

(continued)

(continued)

Drug class	Herb	Potential interaction	Evidence	Recommendations
Antimicrobials				
Erythromycin	*Hypericum perforatum*	*SI* = reduced drug effectiveness	Increases metabolism of erythromycin via induction of CYP3A4, demonstrated in pharmacokinetic trail [7]	Avoid concurrent use to ensure treatment effectiveness [7]
Metronidazole	*Silybum marianum*	*UC* = reduced drug effectiveness	One pharmacokinetic trial showed decreased blood levels of metronidazole. Majority of clinical trials show no interaction with CYP isoforms [8]	Observe patient with concurrent use; however, interaction is unlikely [8, 11]
Voriconazole	*Hypericum perforatum*	*SI* = reduced drug effectiveness	Reduced blood levels of indinavir demonstrated in pharmacokinetic trail via induction of CYP3A4 [7]	Avoid concurrent use to ensure treatment effectiveness [7]
Non-nucleoside transcriptase inhibitors	*Hypericum perforatum*	*SI* = reduced drug effectiveness	Induction of CYP3A4 [7]	Avoid concurrent use to ensure treatment effectiveness [7]
	Ginkgo biloba	*SI* = reduced drug effectiveness	Case report demonstrating reduced effectiveness of Efavirenz causing virologic failure [8]	Mechanism of interaction unknown. Avoid concurrent use. Interaction risk is low for standardized extracts at doses of 240 mg/day or lower [11]
Protease inhibitors	*Silybum marianum*	*UC* = reduced drug effectiveness	Induction of CYP enzymes. No clinical evidence of interactions [8]	Use caution with concurrent use; however, interaction is unlikely [8, 11]
	Hypericum perforatum	*SI* = reduced drug effectiveness	Reduced blood levels of indinavir, demonstrated in pharmacokinetic trail via induction of CYP3A4 [7, 8]	Avoid concurrent use to ensure treatment effectiveness [7]

Barbiturates				
	Galphimia glauca	*OB* = additive effect	Theoretical synergic effect with CNS depressant. In vivo galphimine B been shown to interact with serotonergic transmission [17]	Potential beneficial interaction. Monitoring of patient advised with concurrent use
	Hypericum perforatum	*SI* = reduces drug effectiveness	Induction of CYP enzymes [11]	Avoid concurrent use to ensure treatment effectiveness [18]
	Piper methysticum	*UC* = additive effect	Kava has a synergic effect with CNS depressants [1]	Potential beneficial interaction. May be useful in assisting withdrawal from barbiturates, with drug dose modification. Medical supervision and monitoring of patient advised [18]
	Matricaria recutita	*OB* = additive effect	Theoretical synergic effect with CNS depressant, as apigenin has been found to interact with $GABA_A$ receptors [19]	Potential beneficial interaction. Monitoring of patient advised with concurrent use
	Melissa officinalis	*OB* = additive effect	Theoretical synergic effect with CNS depressants via GABA transmission [20]	Potential beneficial interaction. Monitoring of patient advised with concurrent use
	Passiflora incarnata	*UC* = additive effect	Theoretical synergic effect with CNS depressants. Interacts with $GABA_A$ receptor [21, 22]	Potential beneficial interaction. Monitoring of patient advised with concurrent use
	Scutellaria lateriflora	*UC* = additive effect	Theoretical synergic effect with CNS depressants. $GABA_A$ receptor antagonist [23]	Potential beneficial interaction. Monitoring of patient advised with concurrent use
	Valeriana officinalis	*UC* = additive effect	Theoretical synergic effect with CNS depressants. $GABA_A$ receptor antagonist [24, 25]	Potential beneficial interaction. Monitoring of patient advised with concurrent use
	Withania somnifera	*OB* = additive effect	Theoretical synergic effect with CNS depressants [26]	Potential beneficial interaction. Monitoring of patient advised with concurrent use

(continued)

(continued)

Drug class	Herb	Potential interaction	Evidence	Recommendations
Benzodiazepines				
	Echinacea spp.	*OB* = additive effect	One pharmacokinetic study. Increased oral bioavailability of midazolam [8]	Potential beneficial interaction. Monitoring of patient advised with concurrent use
	Galphimia glauca	*OB* = additive effect	Theoretical synergic effect. In vivo galphimine B been shown to interact with serotonergic transmission [17]	Potential beneficial interaction. Monitoring of patient advised with concurrent use
	Matricaria recutita	*OB* = additive effect	Theoretical synergic effect with benzodiazepines. Apigenin shown to interact with benzodiazepine receptors [19, 27]	Potential beneficial interaction. Monitoring of patient advised with concurrent use
	Hypericum perforatum	*SI* = reduced drug effectiveness	Induction of intestinal CYP3A. One pharmacokinetic trail showed reduced plasma quazepam [1]	Avoid concurrent use to ensure treatment effectiveness [18]
	Piper methysticum	*UC* = additive effect	Kava has a synergic effect with CNS depressants [1]. Case report demonstrated increased lethargy and disorientation when combined with alprazolam [8]	Potential beneficial interaction. May be useful in assisting withdrawal from benzodiazepines, with drug dose modification. Medical supervision and monitoring of patient advised [18, 28]
	Passiflora incarnata	*UC* = additive effect	Theoretical synergic effect with CNS depressants. One case study reported dizziness, hand tremor, throbbing and muscular fatigue (also combined with valerian) [1]	Potential beneficial interaction. Drug dose modification may be needed. Monitoring of patient advised with concurrent use [18]

	Schisandra chinensis	*UC* = increased drug effectiveness	Theoretical synergic effect with CNS depressants. Pharmacokinetic trials reporting Inhibition of CYP enzymes and ABCB1 substrates [11]	Potential beneficial interaction. Clinical significance unconfirmed. Medical supervision needed [18]
	Scutellaria lateriflora	*UC* = additive effect	Theoretical synergic effect with CNS depressants. $GABA_A$ receptor antagonist [23]	Potential beneficial interaction. Monitoring of patient advised with concurrent use
	Valeriana officinalis	*UC* = additive effect	Theoretical synergic effect with CNS depressants. One case study reported dizziness, hand tremor, throbbing and muscular fatigue (also combined with passionflower) [1]	Potential beneficial interaction. Clinical significance unconfirmed. Monitoring of patient advised with concurrent use [18]
	Withania somnifera	*OB* = additive effect	Theoretical synergic effect with CNS depressants [18]	Potential beneficial interaction. Clinical significance unconfirmed. Observe patient with concurrent use [18]
Bronchospasmolytics/bronchodilators				
Theophylline	*Hypericum perforatum*	*OB* = possible reduced drug effectiveness	One case study reported decreased theophylline [8]; however, it has been reported not to have an effect on theophylline kinetics [12]	Interaction unlikely. Monitor patient with concurrent use. Use low-hyperforin extracts such as Ze117 [12]
Cardiovascular drugs				
Cardiovascular drugs (general)	L-Arginine	*OB* = lowers blood pressure	Arginine is generally beneficial for cardiovascular health, yet caution should be exercised when taking in conjunction with heart medications, due to its effects on blood pressure [29]	Observe patient with concurrent use; monitor blood pressure
Anticoagulants (general)	*Eleutherococcus senticosus*	*OB* = increased risk of bleeding	Antiplatelet aggregation compound identified as 3, 4-dihydroxybenzoic acid [30]	Theoretical interaction. Clinical significance unconfirmed. Observe patient with concurrent use [18]

(continued)

(continued)

Drug class	Herb	Potential interaction	Evidence	Recommendations
Digoxin	*Eleutherococcus senticosus*	*UC* = increased drug effectiveness	Once case study reported increased plasma levels of digoxin; however, it had no digoxin toxicity symptoms [31]	Interaction not confirmed. Monitor patient with concurrent use
	Hypericum perforatum	*SI* = reduced drug effectiveness	Pharmacokinetic trials demonstrating decreased digoxin blood concentrations [7, 8]	Avoid concurrent use
Hypolipidaemics (simvastatin, atorvastatin)	*Hypericum perforatum*	*UC* = reduced drug effectiveness	Pharmacokinetic trials demonstrated increased LDL with concurrent use of simvastatin and increased LDL and total cholesterol with atorvastatin [7, 8]	Avoid concurrent use
Talinolol	*Ginkgo biloba*	*OB* = additive effect	Pharmacokinetic trials demonstrating increase blood concentration of talinolol with concurrent use [8, 32]	Mechanism of interaction unconfirmed. Clinical implications unclear. Interaction risk is low for standardized extracts at doses of 240 mg/day or lower [11]
	Schisandra chinensis	*UC* = increased drug effectiveness	Pharmacokinetic trials reporting Inhibition of CYP enzymes and ABCB1 substrates [11]	Potential beneficial interaction. Clinical significance unconfirmed. Medical supervision needed [18]
Warfarin and aspirin	*Ginkgo biloba*	*OB* = increased risk of bleeding	An increased bleeding tendency for warfarin and aspirin has been reported in isolated case studies. However, clinical trials have shown no additive effect on platelet aggregation for aspirin, warfarin, clopidogrel and cilostazol [8]	Observe patient with concurrent use; however, interaction is unlikely [8]
Warfarin	*Hypericum perforatum*	*SI* = reduced drug effectiveness	Pharmacokinetic trail and several case studies reported increased warfarin clearance and decrease anticoagulant effect [7, 8]	Avoid concurrent use

Chemotherapeutics				
Chemotherapy (general)	*Eleutherococcus senticosus*	*UC* = reduced treatment side effects	Theoretical synergistic effect, more research is needed	Potential beneficial interaction. Clinical significance unconfirmed. Medical supervision needed [18]
	Ginkgo biloba	*BI* = reduced drug side effects	Induces CYP enzymes [11]	Interaction risk is low for standardized extracts at doses of 240 mg/day or lower [11]
	Rosmarinus officinalis	*UC* = additive effect	Inhibits P-glycoprotein [33]	Clinical significance unconfirmed. Medical supervision needed with concurrent use
	Silybum marianum	*UC* = reduced drug effect	May decrease paclitaxel and doxorubicin metabolism [34]. Based on pharmacological action, may reduce drug toxicity	Clinical significance unconfirmed. Medical supervision needed with concurrent use. Low risk of interaction [11]
	Hypericum perforatum	*SI* = reduced drug effectiveness	Induces CYP enzymes [7]	Avoid concurrent use as may decrease treatment effectiveness [1]
	Withania somnifera	*OB* = reduced drug side effects and enhanced drug effects	In vivo studies reported reduced drug side effects for cyclophosphamide and doxorubicin; enhanced drug effects were found for concurrent use with paclitaxel [26]	Possible beneficial interaction. Medical supervision needed
Cisplatin	*Silybum marianum*	*UC* = additive effect	Based on pharmacological action, may reduce drug toxicity	Potential beneficial interaction. Clinical significance unconfirmed. Medical supervision needed. Low risk of interaction [11]

(continued)

(continued)

Drug class	Herb	Potential interaction	Evidence	Recommendations
Irinotecan	*Hypericum perforatum*	*SI* = reduced drug effectiveness	Decrease plasma concentration of irinotecan; however, it decreased drug side effects [35]	Avoid concurrent use as may decrease treatment effectiveness. Use low-hyperforin extracts [11]
	Silybum marianum	*BI* = reduced drug side effects	Based on pharmacological action, may reduce drug toxicity. Clinical trials show no effect on pharmacokinetics of irinotecan [8]	Potential beneficial interaction. Clinical significance unconfirmed. Medical supervision needed. Low risk of interaction [11]
Dopaminergics				
Levodopa	*Piper methysticum*	*UC* = reduced drug effectiveness	Case report described reduced activity of levodopa. Possible dopamine antagonist [1, 8]	Avoid concurrent use [1]
Opioids				
Dextromethorphan	*Hypericum perforatum*	*SI* = reduced drug effectiveness	Induction of CYP2D2 enzyme [7]	Avoid concurrent use. May reduce treatment effectiveness. Monitor patients
Methadone	*Piper methysticum*	*UC* = additive effect	Kava has a synergic effect with CNS depressants [1]	May increase sedative effect. Unknown clinical significance.
Methadone, pethidine and oxycodone	*Hypericum perforatum*	*SI* = reduced drug effectiveness	Clinical trial reported decreased plasma concentration of methadone [8]. Induces CYP2D2 enzyme [7]	May reduce treatment effectiveness. Methadone patients may have withdrawal symptoms. Monitor patients. Use low-hyperforin extracts [11]
Hormone-based medication				
Oral contraceptives (etinilestradiol and desogestrel, etinilestradiol and norethindrone)	*Hypericum perforatum*	*UC* = reduced drug effectiveness	Induction of CYP3A4 enzymes; however, this effect is not found to occur with low-hyperforin extracts [8, 36]	Avoid concurrent use with high-hyperforin extracts of *Hypericum* [11]
Thyroid hormones	*Withania somnifera*	*OB* = additive effect	Theoretical increase in drug effectiveness [26]	Monitor patients with concurrent use

Hypoglycaemics				
	Eleutherococcus senticosus	*OB* = additive effect	Theoretical based on pharmacological action. In vitro hypoglycaemic action reported [18]	Unknown clinical significance. Monitor patients with concurrent use
Gliclazide	*Hypericum perforatum*	*UC* = reduced drug effectiveness	Pharmacokinetic trial demonstrated increased incidence of hypoglycaemia, with deceased plasma gliclazide [8]	May reduce treatment effectiveness. Monitor patients. Use low-hyperforin extracts such as Ze117 [11]
Immunosuppressants				
	Eleutherococcus senticosus	*UC* = reduced drug effectiveness	Theoretical based on immunostimulant action	Unknown clinical significance. Monitor patients with concurrent use
Cyclosporine	*Hypericum perforatum*	*SI* = reduced drug effectiveness	Clinical trial demonstrated deceased plasma chlorzoxazone [11]	Avoid concurrent use
	Silybum marianum	*UC* = reduced drug effectiveness and side effects	Theoretical based on pharmacological action, may reduce drug toxicity	May reduce treatment effectiveness. Monitor patients. Low risk of interaction [11]
Tacrolimus	*Hypericum perforatum*	SI = reduced drug effectiveness	Clinical trial demonstrated deceased plasma tacrolimus [7]	Avoid concurrent use
	Schisandra chinensis	*UC* = increased drug effectiveness	Pharmacokinetic trials reporting Inhibition of CYP enzymes and ABCB1 substrates [11]	Potential beneficial interaction. Clinical significance unconfirmed. Medical supervision needed [18]
Muscle relaxants				
Chlorzoxazone	*Piper methysticum*	UC = reduced drug effectiveness	Pharmacokinetic trial in which Kava inhibited CYP2E1 [8]	Avoid concurrent use
	Hypericum perforatum	*SI* = reduced drug effectiveness	Clinical trial demonstrated deceased plasma chlorzoxazone [11]	May reduce treatment effectiveness. Monitor patients. Use low-hyperforin extracts [11]

(continued)

(continued)

Drug class	Herb	Potential interaction	Evidence	Recommendations
Nonsteroidal anti-inflammatory drugs (NSAIDS)				
Ibuprofen	*Hypericum perforatum*	*OB*=possible reduced drug effects	Reduction in plasma ibuprofen reported [7]; however, it has been reported not to have an effect on the drugs kinetics [12]	Interaction unlikely [12]. Observe patient with concurrent use. Use low-hyperforin extracts
Proton-pump inhibitors				
Omeprazole	*Ginkgo biloba*	*UC*=reduced drug effectiveness	Pharmacokinetic trial in which ginkgo reduced blood concentrations of omeprazole and omeprazole sulphone [8]	Mechanism of interaction unknown. Observe patient with concurrent use. Interaction risk is low for standardized extracts at doses of 240 mg/day or lower [11]

References

1. Posadzki P, Watson L, Ernst E. Herb–drug interactions: an overview of systematic reviews. Br J Clin Pharmacol. 2013;75(3):603–18.
2. Cheng N, et al. Antioxidant and hepatoprotective effects of Schisandra chinensis pollen extract on CCl4-induced acute liver damage in mice. Food Chem Toxicol. 2013;55:234–40.
3. Bahmani M, et al. Silybum marianum: beyond hepatoprotection. J Evid Based Complementary Altern Med. 2015;20(4):292–301.
4. Abenavoli L, et al. Milk thistle in liver diseases: past, present, future. Phytother Res. 2010;24(10):1423–32.
5. Liu X, et al. Effects of N-acetylcysteine on metabolism of alcohol and its mechanism research. Chin Pharm J. 2006;41(14):1063–6.
6. Seiva FRF, et al. Alcoholism and alcohol abstinence: N-acetylcysteine to improve energy expenditure, myocardial oxidative stress, and energy metabolism in alcoholic heart disease. Alcohol. 2009;43(8):649–56.
7. Russo E, et al. Hypericum perforatum: pharmacokinetic, mechanism of action, tolerability, and clinical drug–drug interactions. Phytother Res. 2014;28(5):643–55.
8. Izzo AA. Interactions between herbs and conventional drugs: overview of the clinical data. Med Princ Pract. 2012;21(5):404–28.
9. Kulkarni SK, Ninan I. Inhibition of morphine tolerance and dependence by Withania somnifera in mice. J Ethnopharmacol. 1997;57(3):213–7.
10. Smilkstein MJ, et al. Efficacy of oral N-acetylcysteine in the treatment of acetaminophen overdose. Analysis of the National Multicenter Study (1976 to 1985). N Engl J Med. 1988;319(24):1557–62.
11. Gurley BJ, Fifer EK, Gardner Z. Pharmacokinetic herb-drug interactions (part 2): drug interactions involving popular botanical dietary supplements and their clinical relevance. Planta Med. 2012;78(13):1490–514.
12. Rahimi R, Abdollahi M. An update on the ability of St. John's wort to affect the metabolism of other drugs. Expert Opin Drug Metab Toxicol. 2012;8(6):691–708.
13. Gleitz J, et al. Anticonvulsive action of (±)-kavain estimated from its properties on stimulated synaptosomes and Na+channel receptor sites. Eur J Pharmacol. 1996;315(1):89–97.
14. Gastpar M. Hypericum extract WS® 5570 for depression: an overview. Int J Psychiatry Clin Pract. 2013;17:1–7.
15. Benjamin J, et al. Inositol treatment in psychiatry. Psychopharmacol Bull. 1995;31(1):167–75.
16. Zhang XY, et al. A double-blind, placebo-controlled trial of extract of Ginkgo biloba added to haloperidol in treatment-resistant patients with schizophrenia. J Clin Psychiatry. 2001;62(11):878–83.
17. Jimenez-Ferrer E, et al. Interaction of the natural anxiolytic Galphimine-B with serotonergic drugs on dorsal hippocampus in rats. J Ethnopharmacol. 2011;137(1):724–9.
18. Sarris J, Wardle J. Clinical naturopathy. An evidence-based guide to practice. 2nd ed. Chatswood: Elsevier; 2014.

19. Viola H, et al. Apigenin, a component of Matricaria recutita flowers, is a central benzodiazepine receptors-ligand with anxiolytic effects. Planta Med. 1995;61(3):213–6.
20. Awad R, et al. Bioassay-guided fractionation of lemon balm (Melissa officinalis L.) using an in vitro measure of GABA transaminase activity. Phytother Res. 2009;23(8):1075–81.
21. Brown E, et al. Evaluation of the anxiolytic effects of chrysin, a Passiflora incarnata extract, in the laboratory rat. AANA J. 2007;75(5):333–7.
22. Zanoli P, Avallone R, Baraldi M. Behavioral characterisation of the flavonoids apigenin and chrysin. Fitoterapia. 2000;71 Suppl 1:S117–23.
23. de Carvalho RSM, Duarte FS, de Lima TCM. Involvement of GABAergic non-benzodiazepine sites in the anxiolytic-like and sedative effects of the flavonoid baicalein in mice. Behav Brain Res. 2011;221(1):75–82.
24. Muller CE, et al. Interactions of valerian extracts and a fixed valerian-hop extract combination with adenosine receptors. Life Sci. 2002;71(16):1939–49.
25. Benke D, et al. GABA (A) receptors as in vivo substrate for the anxiolytic action of valerenic acid, a major constituent of valerian root extracts. Neuropharmacology. 2009;56(1):174–81.
26. Braun L, Cohen M. Herbs & natural supplements: an evidence-based guide. 3rd ed. Sydney: Elsevier; 2010.
27. Salgueiro JB, et al. Anxiolytic natural and synthetic flavonoid ligands of the central benzodiazepine receptor have No effect on memory tasks in rats. Pharmacol Biochem Behav. 1997;58(4):887–91.
28. Malsch U, Kiese M. Efficacy of kava-kava in the treatment of non-psychotic anxiety, following pretreatment with benzodiazepines. Psychopharmacology (Berl). 2001;157:277–83.
29. L-arginine. Review of natural products. Facts & comparisons [database online] (2010). Wolters Kluwer Health Inc.: St. Louis
30. Yun-Choi HS, Kim JH, Lee JR. Potential inhibitors of platelet aggregation from plant sources, III. J Nat Prod. 1987;50(6):1059–64.
31. Izzo AA, et al. Cardiovascular pharmacotherapy and herbal medicines: the risk of drug interaction. Int J Cardiol. 2005;98(1):1–14.
32. Unger M. Pharmacokinetic drug interactions involving Ginkgo biloba. Drug Metab Rev. 2013;45(3):353–85.
33. Fasinu P, Bouic P, Rosenkranz B. An overview of the evidence and mechanisms of herb-drug interactions. Front Pharmacol. 2012;3.
34. Alsanad SM, Williamson EM, Howard RL. Cancer patients at risk of herb/food supplement–drug interactions: a systematic review. Phytother Res. 2014;28(12):1749–55.
35. Goey AKL, Beijnen JH, Schellens JHM. Herb–drug interactions in oncology. Clin Pharmacol Ther. 2014;95(4):354–5.
36. Madabushi R, et al. Hyperforin in St. John's wort drug interactions. Eur J Clin Pharmacol. 2006;62(3):225–33.

Index

D. Camfield et al. (eds.), *Evidence-Based Herbal and Nutritional Treatments for Anxiety in Psychiatric Disorders*, DOI 10.1007/978-3-319-42307-4

MIX
Papier aus verantwortungsvollen Quellen
Paper from responsible sources
FSC® C105338

If you have any concerns about our products,
you can contact us on
ProductSafety@springernature.com

In case Publisher is established outside the EU,
the EU authorized representative is:
Springer Nature Customer Service Center GmbH
Europaplatz 3, 69115 Heidelberg, Germany

Printed by Libri Plureos GmbH
in Hamburg, Germany